运用 CRISPR-Cas 系统靶向突变型 KRAS 肿瘤的新策略及研究进展

孙美艳　李淼　著

U0038793

吉林大学出版社

·长　春·

图书在版编目（CIP）数据

运用 CRISPR-Cas 系统靶向突变型 KRAS 肿瘤的新策略及研究进展 / 孙美艳 , 李森著 . -- 长春 : 吉林大学出版社 , 2021.3
　　ISBN 978-7-5692-8050-0

　　Ⅰ . ①运… Ⅱ . ①孙… ②李… Ⅲ . ①肿瘤－治疗学
Ⅳ . ① R730.5

中国版本图书馆 CIP 数据核字 (2021) 第 028820 号

书　　名　运用 CRISPR-Cas 系统靶向突变型 KRAS 肿瘤的新策略及研究进展
　　　　　YUNYONG CRISPR-Cas XITONG BAXIANG TUBIANXING KRAS ZHONGLIU DE
　　　　　XINCELÜE JI YANJIU JINZHAN

作　　者　孙美艳　李　森　著
策划编辑　张文涛
责任编辑　曲　楠
责任校对　赵黎黎
装帧设计　昌信图文
出版发行　吉林大学出版社
社　　址　长春市人民大街 4059 号
邮政编码　130021
发行电话　0431-89580028/29/21
网　　址　http://www.jlup.com.cn
电子邮箱　jdcbs@jlu.edu.cn
印　　刷　长春市昌信电脑图文制作有限公司
开　　本　787mm×1092mm　　　1/16
印　　张　11.75
字　　数　180 千字
版　　次　2022 年 1 月　第 1 版
印　　次　2022 年 1 月　第 1 次
书　　号　ISBN 978-7-5692-8050-0
定　　价　55.00 元

序

　　肿瘤严重威胁着人类的身体健康和生命。2020年的最新数据显示，癌症是全球第二大死亡原因，其发病率正呈现年轻化趋势。值得庆幸的是，随着科学技术的发展，虽然癌症的发病率呈上升趋势，但所有年龄段的死亡率几乎都在下降，总体五年存活率也在增加。医药领域对于癌症理解的提升以及对于癌症治疗新方法的不断探索功不可没。目前，治疗癌症的主要手段包括外科手术、放疗、化疗、分子靶向疗法和免疫疗法，其中分子靶向疗法及免疫疗法在临床上属于创新型治疗方式，近年来取得了重大的突破，为癌症治疗提供了新的策略和方向。

　　基因疗法是一种新兴的分子靶向疗法，是指将外源正常基因导入靶细胞，以纠正或补偿缺陷及异常基因引起的疾病，最终达到治疗目的。近年来，已经有多种基因疗法被欧洲药品管理局（EMA）和美国食品药品监督管理局（FDA）批准用于遗传类疾病和癌症的治疗。中国早在1991年就对B型血友病患者展开了基因治疗临床试验，并于2003年批准获得了世界上第一个基因治疗产品——今又生（Gendicine）用于头颈部癌症的治疗。在此后约20年的时间里，中国在基因疗法领域方面不断取得巨大进展。但值得注意的是，传统的基因治疗技术手段具有一定的弊端，它们通常使用病毒载体，并通过表达外源的治疗性基因来治疗遗传疾病。新兴的基因编辑技术则可以通过精准修复病人自身发生突变的基因来进行疾病的治疗，也因而为基因疗法的发展带来了新的方向。特别是CRISPR-Cas基因编辑系统的发现、在真核生物上的成功应用，以及在疾病治疗上的进一步开发，堪称21世纪生物医药领域的最大成就之一。基于利用CRISPR-Cas基因编辑系统在癌症治疗上的大量研究，一些靶向药物已经进入到临床前研究或者临床试验阶段。这给人类攻克癌症这一重大难题带来了曙光。

《运用CRISPR-Cas系统靶向突变型KRAS肿瘤的新策略及研究进展》一书由吉林医药学院孙美艳和吉林大学李淼教授担任主编，他们专注于肿瘤表观遗传学方向研究，同时与美国俄亥俄州立大学纳米生物技术和纳米医学中心郭培宣课题组长期合作，研究药物体内外的传递系统。本书的其他几位来自吉林医药学院、北华大学及温州大学的作者，均在表观遗传学或癌症靶向药物的研发方面具有丰富的研究经验。

本书聚焦了目前国内外靶向突变型原癌基因KRAS在肿瘤治疗中的研究进展和临床意义，近25%的肿瘤细胞中都会存在KRAS突变。因此，能够特异靶向并敲除该突变基因将会在肿瘤控制或治疗上带来重要的积极作用。此外，本书还详细介绍了CRISPR-Cas系统的探索和发现过程，以及在生物研究和临床上的应用。基因编辑传递系统的开发和外泌体作为传递载体的应用也在本书做了详尽的讲解，同时也呈现了编者们近期的科研成果。

本书的出版将为科研工作者在靶向突变型KRAS肿瘤的研究及治疗，以及CRIPSR-Cas基因编辑系统的科研临床应用方面提供权威、全面的使用参考，使从事基础科学领域和临床医学领域的科研工作者们在对靶向治疗、基因编辑、临床前研究和相关问题的攻克上拥有最新的全面而深入的了解，在推动癌症靶向药物研发事业发展方面作出突出贡献。

美国休斯敦大学药学院　　Bin Guo

前 言

KRAS基因点突变是人类癌症中最常见的基因突变，发生在约25%的人类肿瘤中。有研究表明，35%～40%的大肠癌、25%的肺癌以及约90%的胰腺癌中均存在KRAS基因突变。KRAS是首批被发现的致癌基因之一，作为EGFR信号通路下游最重要的效应因子，KRAS在肿瘤信号转导中发挥重要作用。因此，几十年来研究人员一直试图找到能靶向KRAS的药物。由于在结构上缺乏让小分子或药物结合的靶点，KRAS一度被行业认为"不可成药"。近几年，多个针对KRAS^{G12C}的共价抑制剂陆续被开发，并在临床试验中进行评估。这些进展为打破KRAS突变"无药可治"的传说提供了可能性途径。

目前，针对KRAS基因突变常用策略有直接靶向抑制KRAS基因、间接靶向KRAS基因和联合途径抑制，而间接靶向又可以通过抑制Kras信号转导通路和通过表观遗传调控KRAS基因的表达来实现。直接抑制KRAS是治疗KRAS突变肿瘤的理想方法。2019年，安进等几家公司公布了令人振奋的Ⅰ期临床数据，让业界对KRAS抑制剂重新燃起了希望，这是近20年来靶向KRAS突变基因的最大突破，其中以KRAS^{G12C}抑制剂（如AMG 510，MRTX849，JNJ-74699157)最为突出。尽管已有一些KRAS^{G12C}抑制剂进入Ⅰ期临床研究，且显示出治疗肺癌的潜力。但不可忽视的是，这类药物的疗效有限、对于特定肿瘤应答率低、接受治疗的患者肿瘤不能完全缩小、获得性耐药性高且KRAS^{G12C}抑制剂只对一部分患者有效。因此，目前我们迫切需要研究新策略，利用新技术、新方法来开发针对多种KRAS等位基因突变的切实有效的靶向药物。

随着CRISPR-Cas基因编辑系统的飞速发展，其在各个基础研究领域和临床医学领域已得到广泛的应用。该系统是在细菌和古细菌中发现的一种获得性免疫系统。从该系统的发现到作为一种基因编辑技术在生物体上的研究应用经历了30多年的时间。CRISPR-Cas系统能够精准地编辑靶向序列，实现特定基因的突变、目的序列的插入及定向单碱基突变，使得从基因水平上进行癌症的精准治疗成为可能，多种单基因或多基因遗传病的治疗得已实现，病毒引发的疾病得以一一攻克。CRISPR-Cas基因编辑系统的开发和应用是本世纪医学研究和临床治疗上最重要的研究之一，也是人类攻克各种疾病的希望。利用CRISPR-Cas基因编辑技术靶向突变型KRAS肿瘤来抑制肿瘤的生长和治愈KRAS突变引发的癌症是充满希望并大有可为的。

《运用CRISPR-Cas系统靶向突变型KRAS肿瘤的新策略及研究进展》内容全面、新颖，既体现了国内外运用CRIPSR-Cas系统靶向突变型KRAS肿瘤的最新研究成果，也为在研发和应用中出现的问题提出了解决方法，对针对突变型KRAS肿瘤的靶向疗法给予了全面的总结，充分体现了CRISPR-Cas基因编辑系统在医学领域的光明前景。本书主要分为3个部分，第一部分主要介绍靶向突变型原癌基因KRAS在癌症治疗中的研究进展、常用策略及国内外的发展动态；第二部分主要介绍CRISPR-Cas系统的探索和发现过程、结构组成和作用机理，该基因编辑技术在抗肿瘤治疗中的应用、存在的问题及技术改进方法，以及基因编辑技术在突变型KRAS肿瘤治疗上的新思路；第三部分主要介绍CRISPR-Cas基因编辑系统应用上的一大障碍——传递系统，即如何能特异靶向细胞及基因位点，以及传递系统的种类、开发和选用。

本书的编者队伍汇集了国内在表观遗传学、肿瘤学和遗传学方面的研究学者，他们在各自的领域都有很深的学术造诣，发表了多篇高影响力的文章。他们的参与确保本书客观准确地描述了通过CRISPR-Cas基因编辑技术靶向突变型KRAS肿瘤的国内外的研究进展和最新的研究策略。

如果本书的出版能为广大从事癌症靶向疗法研究和基因编辑技术应用的科研工作者，提供一部既有基础理论背景介绍，又能展示目前国内外的研究现状的专著，也能为我国在癌症领域的研究方向提供一定的指导，将是我们最大的心愿。

在此，对本书撰写和出版过程中给予支持和帮助的同道表示衷心感谢，感谢所有为此付出的人。书中难免有不足之处，请读者多加指正。

孙美艳　李淼

2020年7月 16日

目　录

第二部分   CRISPR-Cas 系统的功能和应用

第三部分　基因编辑传递系统及外泌体的应用

KRAS 靶向治疗在癌症中的研究
进展和临床意义

摘　要

　　原癌基因（proto-oncogene）是指普遍存在于人类或其他动物细胞基因组中的一类基因，在生物进化中属高度保守基因序列，对于控制细胞生长分化以及细胞周期起着重要的调控作用。在环境致癌因素下，原癌基因的结构或调控区发生变异，基因产物增多或活性增强时，使细胞过度增殖，从而形成肿瘤。

　　在众多原癌基因中，RAS基因家族在人类肿瘤中突变概率最高，RAS突变肿瘤占人类所有恶性肿瘤的10%~30%。其中KRAS作为RAS基因家族中的主要亚型，其突变促发人类多种致死性实体瘤，如肺癌、结直肠癌和胰腺癌等。然而，由于KRAS信号通路调控复杂，且在结构上缺乏让小分子或药物结合的靶点，使得尽管目前针对KRAS的靶向治疗思路层出不穷，但能顺利通过临床试验并投入使用的药物和方法寥寥无几。本文主要对KRAS的结构功能、突变结果、调控机制、临床意义以及目前对于其靶向治疗的研究进展进行综述，讨论了KRAS核酸蛋白复合物（Hypa-dCas9-HDAC1-sgRNA$_{KRAS}$）的构建、制备及应用。在sgRNA$_{KRAS}$的引导下，融合蛋白Hypa-dCas9-HDAC1与KRAS启动子区结合，进而HDAC1可以使KRAS启动子区核心组蛋白去乙酰基化、与DNA结合紧密、染色质致密卷曲而达到抑制KRAS的转录表达的目的。这个新策略的KRAS临床意义也在本文中进行了讨论。

　　【关键词】KRAS；结构功能；调控机制；基因突变；靶向药；研究进展

Abstract

Proto—oncogenes are a class of genes ubiquitously expressed in human and other organisms. These genes have been highly conservative in biological evolution and play important roles in controlling cell growth, cell differentiation and cell cycle progression. Upon exposure to carcinogenic factors in the environment, mutations occur and lead to the changes in structure or regulatory regions of proto—oncogenes, which increase the expression level or activity of the proto—oncogene and ultimately lead to increased cell proliferation and the formation of cancer.

Among the many proto—oncogenes, RAS gene family has the highest mutation probability in human tumors. RAS mutant tumors account for approximately 10% ~ 30% of all human malignant tumors. The mutation of *KRAS*, a major subtype of RAS gene family, promotes a variety of fatal solid tumors, such as lung cancer, colorectal cancer and pancreatic cancer. However, despite considerable amount of ideas for the targeted therapy for *KRAS*, due to the complex of *KRAS* signaling pathway and the lack of structural targeting sites for small molecules or drugs to bind, *KRAS* there are few drugs and methods that entered clinical phase. This article mainly reviews the structure and functions of *KRAS*, the outcome of *KRAS* mutations, the mechanism of regulating *KRAS* signaling, the clinical significance and current research progresses of the targeted therapy of *KRAS*. We also discussed the strategy *KRAS* of the assembly and application of the nucleic acid—protein complex （Hypa—dCas9—HDAC1—sgRNA$_{KRAS}$）. Under the guidance of sgRNA$_{KRAS}$, the fusion protein Hypa—dCas9—HDAC1 binds to the promoter region of *KRAS*. HDAC1 can then deacetylate the core histone of *KRAS* promoter region，bind closely to DNA and alter the packing density of chromatin and subsequently inhibit the transcription of *KRAS*. The clinical significance of this novel approach is also discussed.

[Keywords] *KRAS*; structure and function; regulatory mechanism; gene mutation; targeted therapy; research progress

1　*KRAS*基因概述

鼠类肉瘤病毒癌基因（kirsten rat sarcoma viral oncogene，*KRAS*），编码21kD的KRas蛋白，故又称*p21*基因，属RAS原癌基因家族。该家族均为编码细胞内信号传导蛋白类原癌基因，其中与人类肿瘤相关的基因包括*HRAS*、*KRAS*和*NRAS*三种亚型，分别定位在11、12和1号染色体上。*KRAS*编码的KRas蛋白为一种小分子G蛋白，在细胞质中合成，广泛分布于细胞内膜。该蛋白整体呈酸性，是细胞内重要的胶原蛋白、核蛋白，并且具有一些RNA结合模体的特征，整体呈现亲水性[1]。KRas蛋白是EGFR信号通路的重要的下游蛋白，具有GTP酶（GTPase）的活性。

在结构上，KRas蛋白具有催化结构域和高变区（HVR）（图1.1）。催化结构域结合鸟嘌呤核苷酸并激活信号传导，而HVR序列则决定了KRas蛋白如何定位在发生信号传导的细胞膜上，催化域由2个叶组成：第一个叶（残基1—86）包含P环（P-loop）和开关（SwitchⅠ和SwitchⅡ）区域；第二个叶（残基87—171）包含氨基酸变化区域，包括涉及疏水性残基与极性或带电荷残基相互交换的几种变化[2]。第一个叶[3]可以视为效应器叶，因为它包含与效应器交互的所有KRAS组件。第二个是变构叶，它与膜相互作用，并在HVR之外表现出所有的异构体特异性差异。响应于GTP的负载而激活的RAS涉及开关Ⅰ和开关Ⅱ[4]中的大的构象变化，以及相对于膜的重新定位，这促进了效应蛋白的结合。由于在体外测量到RAS的缓慢内在水解速率[5]，信号的失活严重依赖于GAP[6]或其他机制对GTPase活性的增强。在后一种情况下，螺旋3/loop7远离开关Ⅱ与无序到有序的转变有关，当酸性基团（最有可能是膜组分）在远程变构位点[7]结合时，该无序到有序转变将催化Q61残基带入活性位点。RAS突变体水解GTP的能力减弱，无论是固有的还是对GAP的响应，都是活性位点G12、G13和Q61残基突变的致癌性质的原因。了解这些残基在促进催化中所起的关键作用对于靶向*KRAS*药物的研发也至关重要。

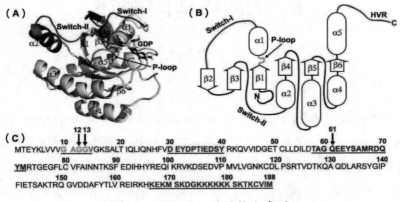

图 1.1　*KRAS*4B 的结构和序列

（A）—与GDP结合的野生型（WT）*KRAS*的晶体结构（PDB ID：4obe），此结构中包含1—169残基；（B）—*KRAS*的二级结构展示；（C）—*KRAS*4B的序列（Uniprot：P01116-2）。颜色标出区域：P环（残基10—14），橙色；开关Ⅰ（残基30—40），红色；开关Ⅱ（残基58—72），蓝色；HVR（残基167—188），绿色。此图片引自参考文献[136]。

*KRAS*基因分为正常和异常两种状态，正常状态称为野生型，异常状态称为突变型。*RAS*基因点突变是人类癌症中最常见的基因突变，发生在10%~30%的人类肿瘤中[8]，其中85%的RAS驱动的癌症是由*KRAS*亚型的突变引起的[9]，且最常见于实体肿瘤。有研究表明[9]，35%~40%的大肠癌，25%的肺癌以及约90%的肺癌中均存在*KRAS*基因突变。*KRAS*基因突变总计有1 848个突变位点，有127个热点突变，但大多数突变发生于第12、13和61密码子。在*KRAS*突变肿瘤中，80%的致癌突变发生在密码子12内，最常见的突变是G12D（41%）、G12V（28%）和G12C（14%）[10]。

　　*KRAS*基因编码两个使用不同外显子4S的剪接变异体，产生*KRAS*4A和*KRAS*4B。*KRAS*4A在C末端另外含有22或23个氨基酸，因此有不同的翻译后修饰和膜定位[11-13]。长期以来，*KRAS*4B一直被认为是主要的异构体，因为它在人类肿瘤[14-15]中普遍高表达。然而，最近发现*KRAS*4A在癌细胞中广泛表达，并且在大肠癌[16]中的表达水平与*KRAS*4B相当。此外，在小鼠模型中*KRAS*4A或*KRAS*4B的缺失可导致对肺癌发生的抵抗效果，这表明肿瘤的启动需要这两种异构体[17]。这两种异构体在肿瘤微环境中也可能有特定的作用，*KRAS*4A的表达提高了对应激环境（如缺氧）的适应能力，而*KRAS*4B在干细胞和祖细胞中均有表达。肿瘤可以通过剪接来适应在压力时期表达*KRAS*4A [17]。这些最近的研究重新关注了*KRAS*4A在肿瘤发生中的作用，并改变了抑制*KRAS*的视角，因此*KRAS*4A现在也需要被重视起来。

　　正常生理情况下，当EGFR或其他酪氨酸激酶受体（RTK）在胞外信号分子的刺激下激活后，形成自磷酸化位点供Grb_2/Sos（Growth factor receptor-bound protein 2/Son of Sevenless）接头蛋白的SH_2（Src-homology 2）结构域特异性识别，后者进一步使KRas蛋白从与GDP结合的无活性形式转变成与GTP结合的有活性形式，继续激活RAF-MAPK及PI3K/AKT等信号通路中的下游蛋白，同时GTP水解成为GDP后KRas迅速失活。通过KRas在激活态与失活态之间的不断切换最终实现对细胞增殖、凋亡、代谢及血管生成的调节。当*KRAS*发生突变时，GTP酶活性降低，在无EGFR活化信号刺激下使其仍处于与GTP结合的持续激活状态，持续激活下游的信号，导致细胞的无序生长、增殖，从而导致肿瘤的发生（图1.2）。

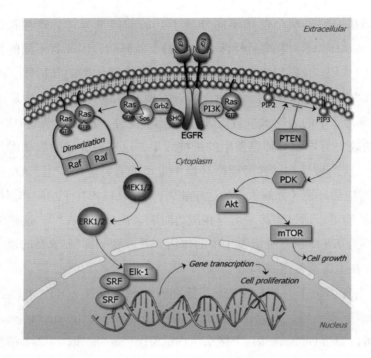

图 1.2 Ras 信号通路

此图片引自参考文献[137]。

因此，我们常把KRas蛋白形容成一个二元双向开关，在信号转导过程中持续的在激活形式和未激活形式之间发生构象变换。这种开关机制高度保守，在GDP/GTP结合蛋白中，可以观察到多种细胞的生长因子、异三聚体G蛋白和大量具有不同生物学功能的小GTP酶。在细胞中存在着一些专门控制小G蛋白活性的小G蛋白调节因子，有的可以增强小G蛋白的活性，如鸟苷酸交换因子（guanine nucleotide exchange factors，GEFs），有的可以降低小G蛋白活性，如GTP酶活化蛋白（GTPase activating protein，GAP）和鸟苷酸解离抑制因子（Guanine nucleotide dissociation Inhibitor，GDI）[18]。因此，靶向这些调节KRas活性的蛋白也为针对*KRAS*突变的治疗性研究提供了间接策略。

2　KRas蛋白的主要作用途径

KRas蛋白是许多细胞内信号转导途径的下游蛋白，尤为重要的是参与控制细胞生成的PI3K–AKT–mTOR信号通路，以及控制细胞增殖的Ras–RAF–MAPK信号通路（如图1.2所示）。受体酪氨酸激酶（RTK）中发生磷酸化的酪氨酸对含有SH$_2$结构域的信号分子具有很高的特异性亲合力，可以看成这类信号分子的固定"泊位"，并触发下游信号传导的级联反应。在此级联反应中，KRas蛋白具有十分重要的作用。了解KRas作用的信号通路有助于通过对上下游的某个重要节点设障，最终拦截KRas激活的信号通路。

当RTK未被活化时，KRas始终与GDP结合，也保持失活状态。当生长因子与其细胞膜受体结合后，促进受体二聚体化，此时胞内区激酶发生活化。活化的激酶必须继续活化KRas蛋白，才能使信号下传。此时，细胞中的KRas蛋白在GEFs的帮助下，把静息时所结合的GDP置换为GTP，KRas因此被活化。活化的KRas参与信号传递。随着信号传递过程的完成，KRas也必须失去活性。由于KRas蛋白具有GTP酶的活性，在GAP的帮助下，KRas可将自身结合的GTP水解为GDP，结合了GDP的KRas则又重新进入失活状态。作为信号分子，KRas之所以能把生长因子的信号继续下传，Grb$_2$和Sos功不可没。这两种蛋白被称为接头蛋白。Grb$_2$为一种胞质游离性蛋白，同时含有SH$_2$和SH$_3$两个结构域，当RTK发生磷酸化后，一方面通过Grb$_2$分子SH$_3$结构域与RTK上的受体结合，另一方面通过Grb$_2$的SH$_3$结构域迅速招募另一信号分子Sos并与之结合，形成RTK/ Grb$_2$/Sos复合蛋白（图2.1）。突变体*KRAS*常伴有蛋白结构改变，使GTP与KRas结合更加牢固，因此，KRas信号通路持续活化，肿瘤细胞因而也被"锁定"在生长与增殖状态。

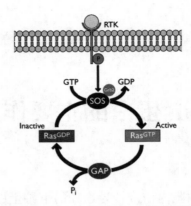

图 2.1 通过 RTK–Grb$_2$–Sos–Ras 通路调控 Ras 活性

此图片引自：https://www.cytoskeleton.com/blog/kras–sos–inhibitor–news

3　*KRAS*基因突变及其临床意义

3.1　常见 *KRAS* 基因突变的分型及分子机制

　　*KRAS*每个亚型突变都表现出对特定癌症类型的优先偶联，每个异构体都可表现出密码子突变和氨基酸替代偏向，这些突变偏向中的许多并不是由于暴露于诱变剂的差异，有可能与潜在或表观的遗传机制以及蛋白质异构体的特异性差异有关。

　　基因毒性物质被认为是导致*KRAS*突变的罪魁祸首。经典的化学致癌研究表明，甲基亚硝基脲在各种癌症类型中多以*KRAS*密码子12的第二个碱基为靶点，产生G12D突变[19-21]。*KRAS*突变模式大多由密码子12或13的第二碱基G-A转换的43%的突变主导，导致G12D或G13D突变。少部分突变为第二个碱基的G-T颠倒置换以产生G12V。*KRAS*突变和剪接变异体是许多癌症类型的遗传驱动因素，包括结直肠癌（CRC）、胰腺导管腺癌（PDAC）、肺腺癌（LUAD，非小细胞肺癌的一个亚型）、黑色素瘤和某些血液系统肿瘤（图3.1）。很大比例的LUAD（～32%）、PDAC（～86%）和CRC（～40%）是由KRAS第12位密码子突变驱动的[21-23]。

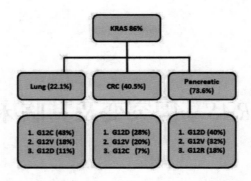

图 3.1 *KRAS* 常见点突变在肺癌、结直肠癌和胰腺癌中的发生概率

此图片修改自参考文献[138]。

3.2　临床意义

3.2.1　肺癌

肺癌占所有癌症相关死亡的约18%，是全球癌症相关死亡的主要原因。它主要包括两种亚型，小细胞肺癌和非小细胞肺癌（NSCLC），后者占肺癌的80%以上[24]。有20%～30%的NSCLC患者存在*KRAS*基因突变。其中约45%的突变是由第12密码子G→T产生G12C引起的[139]，导致KRas蛋白持续激活进一步引起肿瘤的发生（图3.2）。*KRAS*基因突变会导致肺癌患者对EGFR-TKIs产生耐药，对其突变的检测可辅助临床医生筛选受益于EGFR-TKIs的非小细胞肺癌患者。《非小细胞肺癌临床实践指南》（V2.2011）明确指出：当*KRAS*基因发生突变时，不建议使用EGFR-TKIs靶向治疗药物[25]。

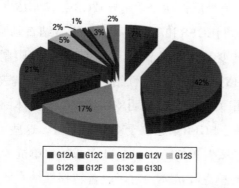

图 3.2　NSCLC 中 *KRAS* 位于 12 或 13 密码子第二个碱基的突变的发生概率

此图片引用自参考文献[140]，数据分析来源自COSMIC（癌症中的体细胞突变目录）数据库。

3.2.2　结直肠癌

*KRAS*基因也是结直肠癌中突变频率最高的基因，*KRAS*基因突变发生于早期腺瘤向中期腺瘤转变阶段，可能是大肠腺恶变的始动基因，其不同的突变类型与结直肠癌的分期及预后相关。G13D突变体出现在25%的*KRAS*驱动的结直肠癌中，而在*HRAS*或*NRAS*中很少观察到。其结构表现为一个开放的活动位点，调整了D13主链扭转角，并具有断开的开关区域离子。在与GDP结合的*KRAS*[G13D]中，A59被放置在Mg2结合位点，使得*KRAS*[G13D]具有破坏核苷酸结合口袋稳定的独特特征[26]。

大多数*KRAS*[G12C]突变型非小细胞肺癌（NSCLC）患者在临床上受益于选择性*KRAS*[G12C]抑制。而具有相同突变的结直肠癌（CRC）患者与NSCLC患者不同，*KRAS*[G12C] CRC模型具有较高的基础RTK激活，并且对生长因子刺激有反应。在CRC系中，*KRAS*[G12C]抑制作用比NSCLC细胞诱导更高的磷酸ERK反弹。尽管几个RTK的上游激活会干扰*KRAS*[G12C]阻滞，但目前已有研究表明，EGFR信号传导是CRC对*KRAS*[G12C]抑制剂耐药的主要机制[28]。EGFR和*KRAS*[G12C]的组合靶向在CRC细胞、患者衍生的类器官和异种移植物中非常有效，这表明治疗CRC患者的新治疗策略。*KRAS*[G12C]抑制剂在NSCLC和CRC中的疗效是谱系特异性的。RTK依赖和信号反弹动力学是导致CRC对$KRAS^{G12C}$抑制的敏感性或抗性的原因，应同时抑制EGFR和$KRAS^{G12C}$，以克服结直肠肿瘤对$KRAS^{G12C}$阻断的耐药性[28]。这种转变是高度调节的，生理反馈回路限制了KRas激活的持续时间[27]。此外，$KRAS$突变还与转移性结直肠癌治疗中抗表皮生长因子受体单克隆抗体的耐药性相关，有证据表明KRas和EGFR受体酪氨酸激酶家族之间存在相互作用[28]。由于EGFR家族位于KRas的上游，这些RTK的失活可以降低KRas的激活。使用西妥昔单抗（Cetuximab）或帕尼单抗（Panitumumab）等抗表皮生长因子受体的单克隆抗体，对于改善转移性结直肠癌和野生型$KRAS$等位基因患者总体生存率有一定作用，但这些抗体对$KRAS$突变肿瘤没有影响。这些临床试验的结果导致西妥昔单抗和帕尼单抗被批准用于治疗缺乏$KRAS$突变的转移性大肠癌。此外，EGFR酪氨酸激酶抑制剂（TKIs），如厄洛替尼（erlotinib）和吉非替尼（gefitinib），被批准用于治疗EGFR突变的NSCLC，但在$KRAS$突变的NSCLC[29-32]中作为单一疗法无效。

3.2.3 胰腺癌

胰腺癌中最常见的是$KRAS^{G12D}$突变，这导致了$KRAS$表达GTPase的显性活性形式。然而，$KRAS$突变如何促进胰腺癌的发生机制尚不清楚。数据显示，在小鼠模型中，在肿瘤发生的早期，诱导致癌基因$KRAS^{G12D}$可在组织损伤后可逆地改变正常的上皮分化，从而导致癌前病变。$KRAS^{G12D}$在已建立的前驱病变和进展为癌症的过程中失活，会导致病变的消退，表明$KRAS^{G12D}$是肿瘤细胞生存所必需的。值得注意的是，在癌变的所有阶段，$KRAS^{G12D}$上调了Hedgehog信号、炎症通路和几条已知介导上皮细胞与其周围微环境之间旁分泌相互作用的通路，从而促进了在胰腺癌中起关键作用的纤维炎症基质的形成和维持。有研究数据证实，上皮$KRAS^{G12D}$影响多种细胞类型以驱动胰腺肿瘤的发生，并且对于肿瘤的维持是必不可少的[33]，因此，我们认为抑制$KRAS^{G12D}$或其下游效应器可能为胰腺癌的治疗提供一种新的方法。

4　国内外发展动态

经过几十年来研究人员的不懈努力，新的研究思路层出不穷，KRAS癌蛋白的共价抑制剂近些年也已经被陆续开发。尽管有些思路在临床试验中没有得到很好地反馈，但是也为我们的研究提供了宝贵的经验。

4.1　KRas 可以被"沉默"

Sunita Shankar等人[34]通过免疫共沉淀技术和质谱分析方法，筛选了细胞内与KRas相互作用的蛋白，发现Argonaute 2（AGO_2）在RNA介导的基因沉默中起着重要的作用。其作用机制为与KRas在内质网膜上共定位，AGO_2通过其N端结构域与KRas相互结合，对突变*KRAS*依赖的癌细胞增殖起到至关重要的作用（图4.1）。在体外细胞实验中研究发现，AGO_2似乎促进了KRas对细胞的促癌转变，突变*KRAS*和AGO_2相互作用会让突变*KRAS*的细胞表现出更强的促癌效果。通过对KRas和其他蛋白的相互作用的研究，以及探索其具体功能研究，将帮助我们找到新的药物靶点，作为癌症药物治疗上的新突破口。

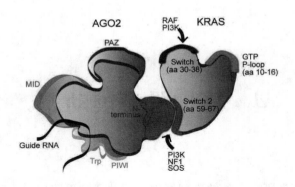

图 4.1　AGO_2 的 N 末端域与 RAS 中的 switch Ⅱ 域相互作用的示意图

此图片修改自参考文献[34]。

4.2　给 $KRAS^{G12C}$ 一个 "刹车"

Shipman 等人[35]设计出一个新型强效抑制剂ARS-853，特异靶向$KRAS^{G12C}$的结合口袋与交换口袋，从而抑制住$KRAS^{G12C}$的生物活性，抑制住其促肿瘤的能力。通过质谱分析手段检测了$KRAS^{G12C}$的生物活性，并通过高分辨率晶体结构分析了ARS-853与$KRAS^{G12C}$的结合能力（图4.2）。研究人员还发现，在多个$KRAS^{G12C}$表达的肺癌细胞内，使用ARS-853能显著降低GTP结合KRAS的水平，还降低了KRas的磷酸化水平以及抑制KRas与下游信号分子的相互作用[35]。多项研究证明了ARS-853诱导癌细胞凋亡、能抑制肿瘤细胞增殖，并通过外源表达$KRAS^{G12C}$能恢复细胞生长与增殖，并进一步证明了ARS-853对$KRAS^{G12C}$的特异性。

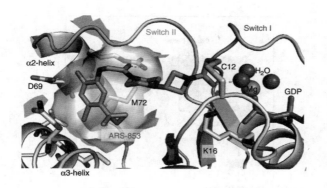

图 4.2　与 *KRAS*^{G12C} 结合的 ARS−853 的晶体结构

Switch Ⅱ 口袋中的关键氢键和疏水相互作用在图片中被强调了出来。图片修改自参考文献[108]。

4.3　首次鉴定出抑制 *RAS* 癌基因的小分子

Premkumar 博士团队[36]鉴定出首个小分子能够同时抑制 *RAS* 癌基因激活的不同信号通路。这个被称作 rigosertib 或 ON-01910.Na 的小分子作为一种蛋白−蛋白相互作用抑制剂发挥作用，阻止 *RAS* 与将正常细胞变成癌细胞的信号蛋白（包括 RAF 和 PI3K 等）相结合（图4.3）。研究人员开展结构学实验，证实了 rigosertib 的这个作用机制，并且证实这种靶向作用机制有潜力用于治疗几种由 *RAS* 癌基因驱动的癌症。Rigosertib 的作用机制代表着一种攻击无药可靶向的 *RAS* 癌基因的新策略。

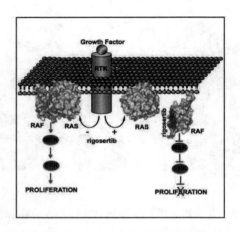

图 4.3 Rigosertib 的作用机制

此图片引用自参考文献[36]。

4.4 PKC 可以调节 KRas 上的法尼酰——静电开关

Trever[37]等人将KRas与质膜（PM）通过法尼酰化结合在一起，与相邻的多基序列一起工作，发现S181蛋白激酶C（PKC）磷酸化可以在多基区内促进KRas与PM的快速解离，并与胞内膜结合，包括线粒体外膜。PKC激动剂以S181依赖的方式促进致癌KRas转化的细胞凋亡。KRas在181位含有磷酰胺残基，通过一种途径诱导细胞凋亡需要BCL-XL。PKC激动剂bryostatin-1以S181依赖的方式抑制致癌KRas转化的细胞的体外和体内生长。实验数据表明，KRas的功能直接受到PKC的调节，并提出了一种用刺激S181磷酸化的药物治疗KRas依赖性肿瘤的方法。

4.5 靶向 ACSL₃ 治疗肺癌的新靶点

Mahesh等人[38]对肺癌中的*KRAS*进行了研究，发现ACSL₃（Acyl-CoA

Synthetase Long Chain Family Member 3，酰基辅酶A合成酶长链家族成员3）介导的*KRAS*活性对于肺癌细胞存活至关重要，抑制ACSL₃就会引起肺癌细胞死亡。ACSL₃的酶活性是突变的*KRAS*基因促进肺癌形成所需要的一个重要条件，进一步研究表明ACSL₃的催化底物——脂肪酸在肺癌中扮演重要角色也成了一个行之有效的新思路。

4.6 基于小分子化合物的"协同致死化学筛选"体系的建立

刘明耀教授及团队成员揭示了*KRAS*突变肿瘤的分子特性以及有效治疗*KRAS*突变肿瘤的临床新策略[39]。共同建立了规模性小分子化合物、临床药物及药物组合筛选体系。研究发现，联合PLK1激酶抑制剂和ROCK激酶抑制剂可特异性激活*KRAS*突变细胞中*p21*的抑癌功能，促发有丝分裂压力，从而有效并特异性地抑制*KRAS*突变细胞生长。该研究系统证实了*KRAS*突变肿瘤对有丝分裂压力的敏感性，首次揭示了*KRAS*基因与*CDKN*1A基因（编码p21蛋白）二者之间的依赖性关系，研究成果为*KRAS*突变肿瘤的治疗提供了新的靶向及有效的临床治疗策略。

4.7 p110位点的发现

Feng Huizhong等人通过对蛋白质结构的计算分析，确定了$KRAS^{G12D}$上一个假定的小分子结合位点[40]，由于它与脯氨酸110相邻，因此称之为p110位点。通过微量热电泳法、热位移法和核磁共振波谱法证实了一种化合物，命名为*KRAS*变构配体KAL-21404358。KAL-21404358不与p110位点的4个突变体结合，削弱了$KRAS^{G12D}$与B-Raf的相互作用，破坏了RAF-MEK-ERK和PI3K-AKT信号通路（图4.4）。这些发现提示p110位点是$KRAS^{G12D}$的小分子变构抑制剂的潜在结合位点。p110位点位于变构叶中，与功能P环、开关Ⅰ和开关Ⅱ区域相反，这些区域构成了GTP水解的活性位点和效应蛋白的相互作用位点，包括Raf、PI3K和GAP，导致$KRAS^{G12D}$信号活性中断。微量热泳（MST）分析表明，这些类似物的结合亲和力有所提高，但它们破坏$KRAS$-RAF相互作用的能力并未增强。这一点还有待进一步研究，特别是利用结构生物学的方法。综上所述，这些发现表明p110位点是一个潜在的针对致癌$KRAS$蛋白的变构调节位点。KAL-21404358是这个位点的第一个小分子候选者。这为发现$KRAS^{G12D}$的小分子变构抑制剂提供了新的策略。

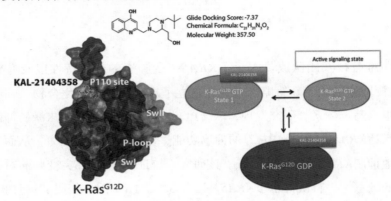

图 4.4　KAL-21404358 的结构及作用机制

此图片引用自参考文献[141]。

　　以上我们汇总了近十年来出现过的比较有代表意义的几种靶向$KRAS$的新策略，然而真正能进入临床试验并取得良好反馈的治疗方案却少之又少。最近随着FDA批准了一种等位基因特异性共价抑制剂AMG 510的临床研究快速通道，临床批准的突变型选择性$KRAS$疗法现已近在眼前。界内对$KRAS$的靶向治疗又燃起了新的希望，下面我们将对目前取得重大进展的几种策略进行逐一综述。

5　目前针对*KRAS*基因突变常用策略

*KRAS*是首批被发现的致癌基因之一，作为EGFR信号通路下游最重要的效应因子，*KRAS*在肿瘤信号转导中发挥重要作用。因此，几十年来研究人员一直试图找到能靶向它的药物。由于在结构上缺乏让小分子或药物结合的靶点，*KRAS*因此一度被行业认为"不可成药"，经过几十年持续不断的研究，*KRAS*^{G12C}癌蛋白的共价抑制剂近些年已经陆续开发了出来，并在临床上进行了试验和评估，为打破*KRAS*突变"无药可治"传说提供了希望。

5.1　直接靶向抑制 *KRAS* 基因

直接抑制*KRAS*是治疗*KRAS*突变肿瘤的理想方法。我们重点介绍直接靶向RAS的最新进展，包括Switch-Ⅱ突变选择性共价抑制剂和PAN-RAS抑制剂的开发。开发突变体特异性KRAS（KRAS^{G12C}）Switch-Ⅱ共价抑制剂的努力正在进展。

Ostem等人首先在突变的*KRAS*^{G12C}蛋白中发现了Switch-Ⅱ后面的一个新的变构结合口袋，称为Switch-Ⅱ口袋[41, 107]。他们开发出第一系列不可逆靶向*KRAS*^{G12C}的化合物。这些化合物以GDP结合状态与*KRAS*^{G12C}结合，阻断Sos催化的核苷酸交换，阻断*KRAS*^{G12C}与Raf的结合。值得注意的是，这些化合物只在GDP结合状态下与*KRAS*^{G12C}结合，因此需要*KRAS*^{G12C}首先进行GTP水解。大约75%的*KRAS*^{G12C}在稳定状态下是GTP结合的，但*KRAS*^{G12C}在常见的致癌突变中具有最高水平的固有GTPase活性，因此容易受到共价攻击。由于*KRAS*不是

$KRAS^{G12C}$中的突变具有较低的固有GTP水解率，因此，尚不清楚通过这些其他突变形式中的类似方法来靶向Switch-II口袋是否会成功。这一发现突出了Switch-II口袋的动态性质，提供了概念验证证据，证明RAS的两种核苷酸结合状态都可以作为抑制剂的靶点。

2019年，安进等公司公布了令人振奋的I期临床数据，让业界对$KRAS$抑制剂重新燃起了希望，这是近二十年来靶向$KRAS$突变基因的最大的突破。其中以$KRAS^{G12C}$抑制剂（如AMG 510，MRTX849，JNJ-74699157）最为突出。尽管已有一些$KRAS^{G12C}$抑制剂进入I期临床研究，且显示出了治疗肺癌的潜力，但不可忽视的是，这类药物的疗效有限：接受治疗的患者肿瘤不能完全缩小，且$KRAS^{G12C}$抑制剂只对一部分患者有效。

5.1.1　AMG 510

随着2019年美国FDA批准了$KRAS^{G12C}$抑制剂AMG 510在NSCLC中的研发快速通道，临床批准的突变型选择性$KRAS$疗法或将在不久的将来取得重大进展。

AMG 510是临床开发中的第一个$KRAS^{G12C}$抑制剂（图5.1）。在临床前分析中，使用AMG 510治疗导致$KRAS$肿瘤消退，并提高了化疗和靶向药物的抗肿瘤疗效。在免疫能力正常的小鼠中，用AMG 510治疗导致促炎性肿瘤微环境，并且单独以及与免疫检查点抑制剂联合产生持久的治疗效果。治愈的小鼠拒绝了同源$KRAS$肿瘤的生长，这表明针对共有抗原的适应性免疫。此外，在临床试验中，AMG 510在首次给药队列中显示了抗肿瘤活性，并代表了对缺乏有效治疗的患者的潜在转化疗法。

ASCO公布了AMG 510一项I期研究（CodeBreak 100）的试验数据[42]，该研究旨在评估AMG 510治疗局部晚期或转移性$KRAS^{G12C}$突变阳性实体瘤成人患者的安全性、耐受性、药代动力学和疗效。该研究共纳入了35例晚期$KRAS^{G12C}$突变癌症患者，其中14例患有非小细胞型肺癌，19例患有结直肠癌，2例患有其他实体瘤。这些患者均接受了≥2线的治疗方案后发生疾病进展。在29例可评估疗效的患者中（包括10例NSCLC及19例CRC），总体ORR（客观有效率）

为17.24%，DCR（疾病控制率）为79.31%，并且疗效持续长久。同时，Ⅰ期试验的初步结果很有希望，特别是在NSCLC中：在接受960mg目标剂量的13例患者中，7例患者有部分应答（PR），6例患者有稳定的疾病（SD）。结直肠癌的活跃性要小得多：12例患者中只有1例患者有PR，10例患者有SD[43]。值得注意的是，在34例患者中，没有一人表现出剂量限制性毒性或导致停药的不良事件。在临床前模型中，AMG 510有效地抑制了*KRAS*[G12C]细胞系的细胞活力，并诱导了异种移植瘤模型的肿瘤消退[42]。当AMG 510与RAS激活或被RAS激活的蛋白抑制剂（如MEK、AKT、PI3K、SHP2和EGFR家族成员）或免疫疗法[42]联用时，具有协同生长抑制效应。

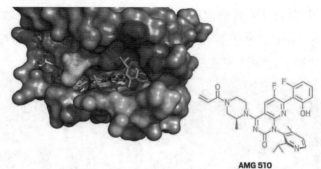

图 5.1　*KRas*[G12C] 与脱氧鸟苷二磷酸（左）和 AMG 510（右）结合

如图5.1所示，黄色区域是AMG 510与半胱氨酸共价连接的区域。粉色区域显示组氨酸被候选药物翻转。右下角为AMG 510化学结构式。此图片引自安进公司官网。

目前，一项针对NSCLC和CRC患者的临床Ⅱ期单臂试验（也是CodeBreak 100试验的一部分）已完成招募，参见参考文献[149]。一项研究多种晚期实体瘤的Ⅰb期药物联用研究正在招募病人（CodeBreak 101）。此外，在NSCLC中开展的全球Ⅲ期确证研究（CodeBreak 200）也已经开始招募。

5.1.2　MRTX849

MRTX849是首批进入临床试验的*KRAS*[G12C]抑制剂之一，被认为是一种高效的、选择性的、共价的*KRAS*[G12C]优化口服抑制剂，具有良好的药物特性，能够选择性地修饰GDP结合的$KRAS^{G12C}$中的突变半胱氨酸12，抑制$KRAS$依赖的信号转导，在体内几乎完全抑制$KRAS$，这为更好地理解该突变在各种癌症中作为致癌驱动因素的作用和指导合理的临床试验设计提供了新的机会（图5.2）。2019年10月公布了MRTX849的Ⅰ/Ⅱ期临床试验数据[44]，在早期的临床研究中（在7例患者中，每天两次服用600mg），5例非小细胞肺癌患者中有3例实现了PR（partial response），2例CRC患者中有1例实现了PR。在临床前模型中，MRTX849有效地降低了$KRAS^{G12C}$细胞系的细胞存活率，并在异种移植模型中引起肿瘤消退。当与EGFR家族抑制剂SHP$_2$、mTOR或细胞周期蛋白依赖性激酶4（CDK$_4$）和CDK$_6$联合使用时，MRTX849表现出协同效应，甚至在MRTX849耐药的肿瘤[45]中也能导致肿瘤消退。在CRISPR筛查中，$NRAS$或Keap1（Kelch Like ECH Associated Protein 1）的缺失导致对MRTX849的耐药性，而SHP$_2$、MYC或mTOR途径基因的缺失进一步使肿瘤对MRTX849敏感。

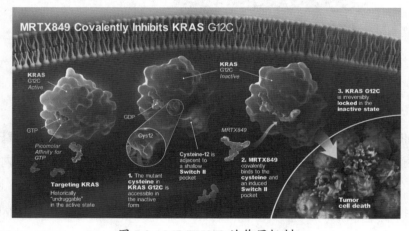

图 5.2　MRTX849 的作用机制

此图片引自MIRATI Therapeutics官网。

MRTX849显示$KRAS^{G12C}$阳性细胞系和患者来源的多种肿瘤类型的异种移植模型中有17例（65%）肿瘤明显消退[45]，在$KRAS^{G12C}$阳性的肺腺癌和结肠腺癌患者中观察到了客观反应。在敏感和部分耐药的非临床模型中，全面的药效学和药物基因组图谱确定了限制抗肿瘤活性的机制，包括$KRAS$核苷酸循环和诱导反馈、重新激活或绕过 $KRAS$ 依赖的途径。MRTX849 与靶向 RTK、mTOR 或细胞周期的药物联合在几种肿瘤模型中显示出增强的反应和显著的肿瘤消退[45]。MRTX849 的发现为患者提供了一个期待已久的选择性靶向 $KRAS^{G12C}$ 的机会。MRTX849 活性的深入表征，反应和耐药机制的阐明，以及有效组合的鉴定，为 $KRAS$ 依赖和这类药物的合理开发提供了新的见解。

MRTX849 对 $KRAS^{G12C}$ 的全面持久抑制为理解 $KRAS$ 作为致癌驱动因子的作用程度提供了独特的机会。此外，观察到 $KRAS$ 在体外和体内对阻断的反应明显不同，这表明在体内模型系统中评价 $KRAS$ 阻断的后果对于理解 $KRAS$ 驱动的肿瘤进展的作用至关重要。在临床试验中，MRTX849 治疗肺腺癌和结肠腺癌患者的部分反应表明，在肿瘤模型中观察到的结果可延伸到 $KRAS^{G12C}$ 阳性的人类癌症[45]。

研究显示，MRTX849 体内治疗导致剂量依赖的 $KRAS^{G12C}$ 修饰，$KRAS$ 通路抑制和抗肿瘤效应[45]。评估 MRTX849 的抗肿瘤活性及其体内药代动力学和药效学特性，可以帮助了解该药的临床应用，并为治疗反应提供洞察力。为了评价 MRTX849 的药效学反应，将药物暴露与靶点抑制联系起来，对移植瘤小鼠口服一定剂量范围的 MRTX849，并在规定的时间点收集血浆和肿瘤。血样分析显示共价修饰的 $KRAS^{G12C}$ 蛋白的比例与 MRTX849 的血浆浓度成正比。随着时间的推移进行评估时，$KRAS^{G12C}$ 的修饰部分在给药后 6h 为 74%，到 72h 逐渐下降到 47%[45]。因此，可以得出结论，尽管血浆中 MRTX849 水平下降，这种延长的药效学效应与 MRTX849 对 $KRAS^{G12C}$ 的不可逆抑制以及 $KRAS^{G12C}$ 蛋白相对较长的半衰期（24 ~ 48h）是一致的。$KRAS^{G12C}$ 的修饰在每天以 30 mg/kg 重复给药 3d 后达到最大，更高的剂量水平在多种肿瘤模型中没有显示额外的 $KRAS^{G12C}$ 修饰[48]。尽管增加了 MRTX849 的剂量和血浆水平，但最大修饰水平不再增加，这表明利用液相色谱-质谱联用（LC-MS）可能无法准确测量 $KRAS^{G12C}$ 的完全抑制，因为肿瘤中存在活性的、非循环的或未折叠的 $KRAS^{G12C}$ 蛋白池。总之，上述研究表明，MRTX849 对 $KRAS^{G12C}$ 的共价修饰呈剂量依赖性增加，$KRAS^{G12C}$ 突变的肿瘤广泛依赖突变的 $KRAS$ 来获得肿瘤细胞的生长和存活，MRTX849 通过 $KRAS^{G12C}$ 依赖的机制产生抗肿瘤活性。

虽然MRTX849在大多数被测试的模型中表现出显著的抗肿瘤反应，但在异种移植组中观察到了从延迟肿瘤生长到完全消退的过程中，机体敏感性上调。由于对MRTX849体外抗肿瘤活性的敏感性与体内模型系统之间缺乏显著相关性，因此有必要进一步研究*KRAS*癌基因在体内肿瘤模型中的依赖性，这是一个更具临床意义的环境。MRTX849在*KRAS*^{G12C}突变的体外癌症模型中显示出显著的抗肿瘤效果，并在大多数实体瘤中显示出显著的消退。然而，临床数据也表明，在不同的肿瘤中，癌细胞对*KRAS*^{G12C}突变存在的生长和存活的依赖程度可能会有所不同，在*KRAS*突变的癌症中观察到的共生基因改变可能会影响直接靶向治疗的反应。进一步观察到，*KRAS*突变发生在不同的癌症中，并且没有单一的共生基因改变可以预测对治疗的反应，这表明了*KRAS*驱动的癌症的遗传异质性。*KRAS*突变细胞对靶基因敲除有非常显著的反应，反应的异质性大小，并且没有明显的共生畸变预测对靶标阻断的抗性[46-47]。综上所述，这些数据进一步说明了*KRAS*突变癌症的异质性和复杂性，并表明目前没有发现二元共生的遗传事件可以预测治疗反应。

MRTX849能够快速而显著地抑制ERK途径调节的转录，如DUSP和spry/spred家族成员，并与ERK和RTK信号的重新激活有关（图5.3）[48]。双特异性磷酸酶DUSP4和DUSP6被MRTX849强烈抑制，并参与ERK1/2的去磷酸化和失活，而Spry家族成员参与RTK、接头蛋白（如Grb_2）的负调控，并可能参与修饰RAS家族的核苷酸交换和效应器结合[49]。

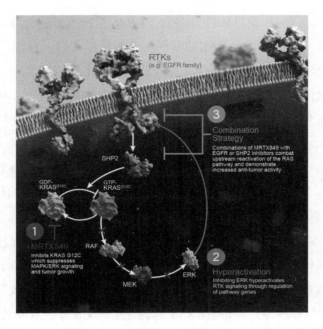

图 5.3 MRTX849 对 RTK 信号通路的调控及与 RTK 抑制剂的联用机制

此图片引自MIRATI Therapeutics官网。

以上两种共价抑制剂，在机制上，研究者发现[50]：AMG 510能抑制ERK的磷酸化；MRTX849能抑制*KRAS*下游的核糖体蛋白S6的磷酸化。二者都可以通过诱导细胞凋亡的方式，抑制细胞的存活。AMG 510和MRTX849，二者都表现出较高的选择性。因为这两种抑制剂，都只能抑制*KRAS*^{G12C}突变细胞的生长。虽然，MRTX849可以在细胞模型和PDX模型中，显著抑制肿瘤的生长，但是，其抗肿瘤的效应差异很大：既可以延迟肿瘤的生长，也可以诱导肿瘤的消退。遗憾的是，目前还没有有效的 biomarker，可以用于预测MRTX849治疗的效果。目前也没有发现，可以预测MRTX849敏感性的基因变异。但是，已经证实，如果细胞内存在细胞周期或mTOR通路相关基因的丢失（包括SHP$_2$和MYC），将有助于MRTX849发挥更好的肿瘤抑制效果。所以，我们认为EGFR/HER2抑制剂：afatinib（阿法替尼）、SHP$_2$抑制剂RMC4550、mTOR抑制剂 vistusertib和everolimus（依维莫司）、CDK$_4$和CDK$_6$抑制剂 palbociclib（帕博西尼），都可以进一步促进MRTX849对于$KRAS^{G12C}$突变细胞的抑制作用。类似现象也发生在AMG 510上：MEK抑制剂、卡铂化疗方案，也都可以增强AMG 510的抗肿瘤反应。AMG 510不仅在免疫缺陷小鼠上进行了实验，还在免疫功能正常的小鼠体内，进行了验证。这种效果依赖T细胞。因为，在免疫缺陷的小鼠体内，虽然肿瘤会消退，但是最终小鼠体内的肿瘤会复发[50]。只有在免疫功能正常的小鼠体内，才能获得持久性治疗的效果。这也提示，免疫系统在介导肿瘤治疗过程中的重要作用。单独使用PD-1疗法或单独采用AMG 510处理，仅获得有限疗效（仅1/10的小鼠出现效果）。联合使用PD-1抗体/AMG 510，能获得显著疗效（9/10的小鼠出现效果）在肿瘤处，AMG 510还能诱导免疫细胞发生浸润，并促进炎性微环境的形成。由于AMG 510促使肿瘤细胞高表达MHC I 类抗原，这使得$KRAS^{G12C}$，再接种到AMG 510治愈的小鼠身上后，无法再形成移植瘤。更有意思的是，用AMG 510处理后，不仅带有$KRAS^{G12C}$的细胞无法形成移植瘤，连带有$KRAS^{G12D}$的细胞也无法形成移植瘤[50]。

5.1.3 ARS-3248 和 LY3499446

$KRAS^{G12C}$共价抑制剂JNJ-74699157（ARS-3248）目前正处于 I 期临床试验，结果尚未公布。以前的两个化合物ARS-853和ARS-1620仅在$KRAS^{G12C}$突变的肿瘤细胞系中抑制细胞生长和抑制MAPK的下游信号。另外一种$KRAS^{G12C}$共价抑制剂LY3499446目前正处于 I / II 期临床试验，作为单一疗法，与CDK4/CDK6或EGFR抑制剂或化疗（多西紫杉醇）联合使用，结果还没有公布。

5.2 间接靶向 $KRAS$ 基因

由于所讨论的共价抑制剂要求$KRAS^{G12C}$处于GDP结合状态，$KRAS^{G12C}$可能会出现耐药性突变，使GTPase活性失效或促进GDP与GTP的鸟嘌呤交换。但众所周知，靶向治疗的耐药性很常见，可能会限制住$KRAS$抑制剂（KRASi）的长期疗效，全面表征KRASi的抗性机制的重要性不言而喻。Joseph Mancias等人[51]建立了目前为止最全面的*KRAS*i蛋白组学库，定量了10 805种蛋白质，最终确定了*KRAS*i与磷脂酰肌醇-3-羟激酶（PI3K），HSP90，CDK4/6和SHP$_2$抑制剂的有效组合。目前，通过等位基因特异性抑制剂直接抑制突变型*KRAS*提供了最佳的治疗途径。针对*KRAS*激活通路或*KRAS*效应通路的治疗，可以与这些直接*KRAS*抑制剂、免疫检查点抑制剂或T细胞靶向方法相结合，以治疗*KRAS*突变的肿瘤。

　　间接靶向*KRAS*的途径需要核苷酸交换、加工、膜定位和效应器结合。改变这些基本步骤中的一个可以用来间接抑制*KRAS*的激活。

5.2.1　抑制 Kras 信号传导通路

　　靶向Kras通路有两种不同的方法：识别具有*RAS*突变的合成致死基因，或靶向酪氨酸激酶受体（例如EGFR家族）和RAS效应通路，即MAPK和PI3K。

　　Kras信号通路下游有RAf-MEK-ERK，PI3K/AKT-mTOR，通过对上下游的某个重要节点设障，最终拦截Kras激活的信号通路也是一种行之有效的思路。*KRAS*突变的肿瘤细胞，MEK下游的ERK对RAF有负反馈作用，只使用MAPK抑制剂，MEK下游的ERK负反馈被抑制，RAF激活后强力激活MEK，导致对MEK抑制剂的快速耐药。所以针对*KRAS*突变的治疗策略是要同时抑制RAF和MEK才能有效阻断Kras的下游信号通路（图5.4）。

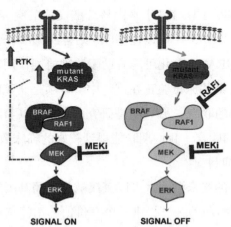

图 5.4　共抑制 MEK 和 RAF 从而阻断 Kras 下游信号通路

此图片引自参考文献[142]。

5.2.1.1　MAPK 通路

5.2.1.1.1MEK抑制剂

目前，有三种针对MEK的变构激酶抑制剂cobimetinib、trametinib和binimetinib临床被批准用于治疗突变实体素瘤。评估MEK抑制剂作为*RAS*突变肿瘤单一疗法的临床试验没有发现任何改善，并且没有MEK抑制剂被临床批准用于治疗*RAS*突变肿瘤[52-54]。MEK抑制剂，与RAF抑制剂相似，会在*RAS*突变的肿瘤中诱导通路反馈，导致对这些肿瘤[55-57]的疗效相对较低。

虽然单药MEK抑制剂在治疗*RAS*突变型肿瘤的临床上已基本失败，但值得注意的是，对于*KRAS*突变的PDAC、CRC和NSCLC，MEK抑制剂的类似临床试验显示没有超过CARE 147，154–156的标准[58]。

由于MEK或RAF抑制剂单一治疗不能为*KRAS*突变肿瘤提供临床益处，这两种抑制剂联合使用的疗效正在临床探索中。由于MAPK通路反馈环的复杂性，靶向MAPK通路的多个节点可导致磷酸化ERK的持续持久抑制（ERK被激活的一种指标，也是MEK的直接靶点；磷酸化ERK通常被用来衡量整个MAPK通路的活性）。事实上，MEK和RAF抑制剂的组合在*RAS*突变肿瘤细胞的临床前模型中显示出协同作用，并阻断了通路的重新激活[59]。此外，MEK和RAF联合治疗的协同效应需要在MEK抑制剂治疗时诱导磷酸化的MEK和GTP结合的RAS。MEK和RAF抑制在具有高水平内核苷酸交换的突变*KRAS*的细胞中观察到最强的协同效应，$KRAS^{G13D}$可以提高GTP结合的RAS水平。这一观察结果表明，MEK抑制诱导的RAF二聚化可能有助于这种协同作用。目前，结合RAF和MEK抑制剂的两个 I 期临床试验正在进行中。一项是研究Belvarafenib（RAF抑制剂）和cobimetinib的联合，另一项是研究曲美替尼（MEK抑制剂）和LXH–254（RAF抑制剂）的联合。我们期盼能得到较好的临床数据。

5.2.1.1.2　ERK抑制剂

抑制ERK级联中的终末激酶，可以直接减少致癌基因的转录输出，并为对MEK或RAF抑制[60-61]耐药的肿瘤提供一个有价值的治疗选择。ERK抑制剂的临床开发滞后于MEK、BRAF单体和PAN–RAF抑制剂的开发。此外，ERK抑制剂治疗*RAS*突变肿瘤的早期临床试验在很大程度上是不成功的。

临床前化合物SCH-772984通过与ERK1/2结合并抑制ERK1/2，同时也诱导构象偏移，阻止ERK1/2通过上游激酶[62-63]磷酸化，作为一种双重机制的ERK1/2抑制剂。用SCH-772984处理RAS突变的癌细胞株可降低磷酸化的ERK水平，并降低细胞增殖[64]。默克公司开发出的MK-8353，与SCH-772984相比具有更好的药代动力学特性。然而，在MK-8353的Ⅰ期单一疗法临床试验中，在登记的160例*KRAS*或*NRAS*突变的26例患者中没有观察到抗肿瘤反应[65]。

GDC-0944在*KRAS*突变肿瘤模型[66]中与Cobimetinib联合使用显示出疗效。尽管临床前异种移植模型显示可以达到导致生长减慢的治疗剂量，但由于患者不能耐受组合[67]，Cobiminib和GDC-0994的Ⅰ期临床试验被终止。

然而，当GDC-0994被评估为单一疗法时，在Ⅰ期临床试验中，14例患有*BRAF*突变CRC或胃癌的患者接受了GDC-0094治疗，其中2例患者有PR，7例患者有SD，5例患者有疾病进展[68]。在14例登记了*KRAS*突变肿瘤的患者中，4例患者实现了SD，10例患者患有进展性疾病[68]。GDC-0994在使用NanoString基因表达的配对肿瘤活检组织中诱导MAPK通路抑制（19%～51%），并且在部分*BRAF*突变的CRC患者中观察到比那些*KRAS*突变的PDAC患者更大的抑制作用[68]。

KO-947目前正处于*KRAS*突变体和BRAF突变体NSCLC的Ⅰ期临床试验中[69]，在临床前模型中有效地降低了磷酸化ERK的水平。观察到持续的反应；磷酸化ERK水平在Kvitro167单剂量后被抑制长达5天。这些特性与所讨论的其他ERK抑制剂不同，提示KO-947可能提供治疗优势。然而，这种磷酸化ERK的持续抑制在患者中可能不是很好的耐受性。

LY3214996，目前正处于Ⅰ期临床试验，是ERK$_1$和ERK$_2$有效和选择性的体外抑制剂[70]（图5.5）。该研究设置了剂量递增组，33例*KRAS*突变型和16例*BRAF*突变型的接受治疗的肿瘤患者中，7例*BRAF*突变患者肿瘤消退，2例SD患者，1例*RAS*突变肿瘤患者SD，而其余患者无明显疾病进展[71]。

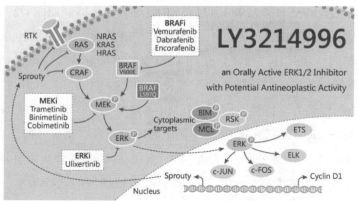

图 5.5　LY3214996 抑制 ERK 通路

此图片引自 Network of Cancer Research 网站。

总体而言，单药 MEK、RAF 或 ERK 抑制剂对 *RAS* 突变肿瘤的治疗效果甚微。因此，这些抑制剂必须与 MAPK 途径的其他抑制剂或本综述中讨论的其他方法联合使用，为每种类型的抑制剂找到最佳组合将是一个挑战。我们认为，等位基因特异性 *KRAS* 抑制剂的出现增加了可用于实现最大途径抑制的潜在组合的数量。

5.2.1.1.3　RAF 抑制剂

从分子机制上来说，活性的 GTP 结合的 *KRAS* 促进 RAF 的二聚化和磷酸化，从而诱导 RAF 激酶活性，并导致 RAF 底物 MEK_1 和 MEK_2 的磷酸化。随着末端激酶 ERK_1 和 ERK_2 的 MEK 磷酸化，磷酸化级联继续进行。ERK 激酶活性既激活促进生长的转录因子，包括 ETS 家族成员，又参与负反馈[72]。该动态过程控制 MAPK 信令级联的持续时间和幅度。ERK 可以通过磷酸化上游组分 Sos 或 CRAF，或通过改变双特异性磷酸酶（DUSP）家族和芽孢蛋白（Sprouty）家族[73-74]的转录来负向抑制 MAPK 信号转导。DUSPs 通过隔离 Sos-Grb_2 使 ERK 去磷酸化，而 SPRY 通过隔离 Sos-Grb_2 抑制受体酪氨酸激酶信号[75]。要有效治疗 *KRAS* 突变肿瘤，必须几乎完全抑制 MAPK 通路。实现这一点的一种策略是使用激酶抑制剂来对抗 MAPK 通路的组成部分，并结合本综述中讨论的其他机制的治疗。

目前，针对 BRAF-V600 和 MEK 的激酶抑制剂已被批准用于 BRAFV600 突变的转移性黑色素瘤，但不适用于 *KRAS* 突变的肿瘤。临床批准的 BRAF-V600 抑制剂，如维莫拉非尼和达普拉非尼，可诱导RAF激酶区域的αC螺旋外移稳定在非活性位置[76]。这些抑制剂有效地抑制RAF单体，但不能用于通过BRAF和CRAF二聚体发出信号的*KRAS*突变肿瘤。此外，在*RAS*突变的肿瘤中，这些抑制剂被证明通过与野生型RAF结合，诱导RAF二聚化以及MEK和ERK的下游磷酸化[77]，反常地激活MAPK通路。矛盾激活依赖于抑制剂结合的模式：在*KRAS*突变肿瘤中，RAF二聚体抑制剂比批准的BRAF-V600抑制剂表现出的矛盾激活要少得多[78]。

5.2.1.1.4　RAF二聚体抑制剂

目前已报道的RAF二聚体抑制剂主要包括AZ-628、Belvarafenib、LY3009120和LXH-254，这些小分子化合物可以将这些小分子化合物可以与RAF结合在Asp-Phe-Gly（DFG）基序列活性位置131—133[79-80]，对RAF单体和二聚体有效（图5.6）。虽然它们也可以促进二聚化，但因为它们可以结合这两个二聚体成分，所以激活互斥反应最小。目前已有报道许多抑制剂作为PAN-RAF抑制剂对*RAS*突变型和*BRAF*突变型肿瘤[81-82]有效。评估LY3009120的Ⅰ期临床试验由于缺乏临床疗效而终止，因为最好的总体结果是SD仅15%[83]。

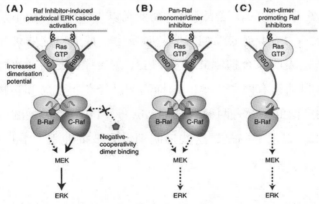

图 5.6　RAF 二聚化对 RAF 抑制剂治疗的影响：克服 RAF 二聚体的困境

如图5.6所示，（A）RAF二聚化可通过在活化的RAS存在下增加RAF的二聚化潜力来影响第一代RAF抑制剂的有效性，从而促进悖论性ERK活化。（B）和（C）为克服RAF二聚体难题，现已开发出对单体和二聚RAF具有相同结合效价并抑制所有RAF家族成员的化合物。RAF单体/二聚体抑制剂可改变αC螺旋位置，以防止/破坏RAF二聚化的药物。RBD即Ras结合域。此图片引用自参考文献[148]。

5.2.1.2　PI3K 途径抑制剂

在所有的KRAS效应中，MAPK通路一直是抑制*KRAS*突变肿瘤的主要焦点。然而另一个效应途径PI3K，也被*KRAS*激活。以下将详细描述PI3K抑制剂的类型以及这些抑制剂治疗*KRAS*驱动的肿瘤的疗效（图5.7）。

有三类PI3K途径抑制剂（图5.7）。目前仅Ⅰ类抑制剂获得了较多有效的数据，从分子机制上来说，该类PI3K被GTP结合的*KRAS*激活后，磷酸化磷脂酰肌醇4，5-二磷酸（PIP_2）生成磷脂酰肌醇-三磷酸（PIP_3），从而将AKT募集到膜上，从而激活mTOR。Ⅰ类PI3K通常由包含RBD的催化亚单位P_{1110}和调节亚单位P_{85}组成的杂化二聚体组成。四个基因（*PI3KCA*、*PI3KCB*、*PI3KCD*和*PI3KCG*）分别编码p110α、p110β、p110γ和p110δ。p110α和p110β亚型普遍表达，而p110γ和p110δ一般只在免疫细胞[84-85]中表达。p110β和p110γ亚型可被G蛋白偶联受体和受体酪氨酸激酶激活[86-87]。通过激活*PI3KCA*突变、AKT扩增或PTEN缺失上调PI3K通路，PTEN编码一种将PIP_3转化为PIP_2的末端磷酸酶[88-89]。PI3K通路突变可以与*KRAS*突变共存，而*KRAS*突变和MAPK通路突变是互斥的，这表明*RAS*突变足以失调MAPK而不是PI3K通路。PI3K通路的激活可在化疗或MAPK抑制时发生，使人对这两种疗法产生抗药性[90]。此外，这表明联合抑制MAPK和PI3K在治疗RAS驱动的肿瘤发生中可能是有效的。目前已有四种Ⅰ类PI3K抑制剂已经获得食品和药物管理局的批准，其中应用广泛的主要有两种：Alpelisib，是p110α特异性的；Copanlisib，是泛Ⅰ类PI3K。很遗憾的是，这些抑制剂没有被批准用于治疗*KRAS*突变的肿瘤。

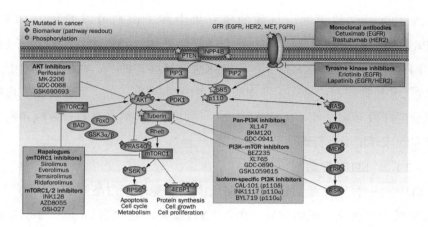

图 5.7　PI3K / AKT-mTOR 信号通路传递和靶向该通路各成分的相关药物

缩写：4EBP1，真核翻译起始因子4E结合蛋白1；BAD，BCL2细胞死亡拮抗剂；CDKN1，细胞周期蛋白依赖性激酶抑制蛋白1；FASLG，Fas抗原配体；FoxO，前叉箱蛋白O；GFR，生长因子受体；GSK3，糖原合酶激酶-3；HIF1，缺氧诱导因子1；INPP4B，Ⅱ型肌醇3，4-双磷酸酯4-磷酸酶；mTORC，mTOR复合体；PDK1，3-磷酸肌醇依赖性蛋白激酶1；PIP$_2$，磷脂酰肌醇（4，5）-二磷酸；PIP$_3$，磷脂酰肌醇（3，4，5）-三磷酸；PRAS40，富含脯氨酸的AKT1底物1；PTEN，磷酸酶和张力蛋白同源物；RPS6，40S核糖体蛋白S6；RSK，90 kDa核糖体蛋白S6激酶。此图片引自参考文献[147]。

　　许多抑制PI3K / AKT-mTOR信号通路中的不同节点的化合物已被开发出来。这些包括PI3K抑制剂根据其选择性可分为泛PI3K抑制剂、双重泛PI3K-mTOR抑制剂和构型特异性PI3K抑制剂，mTOR抑制剂可分为变构抑制剂和mTOR催化抑制剂，而AKT抑制剂包括变构抑制剂和催化抑制剂。

　　RAS同时激活PI3K和MAPK通路，并且存在提供串扰的重叠反馈机制。抑制一条途径可以导致另一条途径的补偿激活。因此，我们认为同时抑制MAPK和PI3K才是行之有效的策略[91]。临床前模型表明，联合抑制PI3K和MEK对*KRAS*突变肿瘤的治疗是有效的[92-93]，并且认为在临床上是可以实现的。然而，在真正的临床试验中，这些抑制剂的组合并不耐受，我们猜测可能是由于毒性减少了剂量[94]。

为了克服这种毒性，目前的研究集中在了识别可以抑制PI3K和/或MAPK的受体酪氨酸激酶。其中一个这样的受体，胰岛素样生长因子1受体（IGF1R），是突变的*KRAS*介导的PI3K激活所必需的[95]。在小鼠模型中，用*KRAS*^{G12C}共价抑制剂代替MEK抑制剂与IGF1R抑制剂linsitinib联合使用，可提高该组合的疗效和耐受性。IGF1R和*KRAS*^{G12C}共价抑制剂组合的有效性和耐受性需要在临床环境中进行评估[95]。

5.2.1.3　SHP$_2$抑制剂

SHP$_2$是一种完全激活MAPK通路所需的非受体蛋白酪氨酸磷酸酶[96]，为首次发现的致癌酪氨酸磷酸酶，由PTPN11编码，在致癌*KRAS*突变驱动的肿瘤中起着不可或缺的作用[97]。SHP$_2$含有两个SH$_2$结构域（N-SH$_2$和C-SH$_2$）、一个催化结构域（PTP）和一个具有两个酪氨酸磷酸化位点的C端尾[98]。SHP$_2$对RAS/ERK信号通路具有促进癌细胞存活和增殖的激活作用[99]。在基底状态下，N-SH$_2$结构域与PTP结构域相互作用，导致PTP活性的自抑制。在刺激细胞后，SHP$_2$通过其SH$_2$结构域到酪氨酸磷酸化生长因子受体或对接蛋白，破坏了这种分子内相互作用，进而导致PTP结构域的暴露，并允许底物进入PTP的催化位点。多受体酪氨酸激酶（RTKs）作用于SHP$_2$，结合生长因子信号促进RAS激活[100]。基因敲除或药理抑制SHP$_2$通过破坏Sos1介导的RAS-GTP负载来破坏致癌RAS/ERK信号和癌症生长[100]。在目前的模型中，SHP$_2$作为支架蛋白，结合Grb$_2$和Sos1，从而增加KRas核苷酸交换[101-102]。SHP$_2$的抑制作用类似于Sos1抑制剂，并通过GTP阻断野生型RAS的负载。*KRAS*突变的肿瘤依赖于SHP$_2$，因为在已建立的肿瘤中抑制SHP$_2$延缓了肿瘤的进展，但不会导致肿瘤的退化[103]。将SHP$_2$锁定在自动抑制构象中的分子的化合物上，发现了SHP$_{99}$对SHP$_2$具有有效的变构抑制作用。在*KRAS*^{G12C}患者衍生的有机物和PDAC和NSCLC的异种移植模型中，SHP$_{99}$与曲美替尼联合使用时可以协同降低细胞增殖。然而，在*KRAS*^{G13D}突变细胞系MDA-MB-213中没有观察到对SHP$_{99}$的敏感性[103]。

RMC-4550是一种高效的选择性SHP$_2$变构抑制剂，可与SHP$_{99}$结合在同一位点，并稳定SHP$_2$的自动抑制构象[104]。RMC-4550治疗减少了临床前模型中的细胞增殖，但这种影响只在 *KRAS* 密码子12突变的细胞中明显，而不存在于13密码子或61密码子突变的细胞中。此外，*KRAS*^{G12C}突变细胞对该化合物的敏感性最高，*KRAS*^{G12D}或*KRAS*^{G12V}突变细胞对该化合物的敏感性较低。这一观察结果表明，每个突变的生化特性决定了KRas活性依赖于鸟嘌呤交换的程度，并且具有升高的内在或GAP介导的水解的突变对SHP$_2$的抑制特别敏感。

SHP$_2$抑制剂与MEK抑制剂联用是目前认为很可能可行的策略（图5.8）。临床候选药物RMC–4630来自RMC–4550[105]，目前处于Ⅰ期单一疗法临床试验和与另一种MEK抑制剂cobimetinib联合进行的Ⅰ/Ⅱ期临床试验。第二种SHP$_2$变构抑制剂JAB–3068，目前处于Ⅰ/Ⅱ期临床试验，结果尚未公布。第三种SHP$_2$抑制剂TNO155正在进行Ⅰ期单一疗法临床试验和与MRTX849联合进行的Ⅰ/Ⅱ期临床试验。这些研究的结果还没有发表。

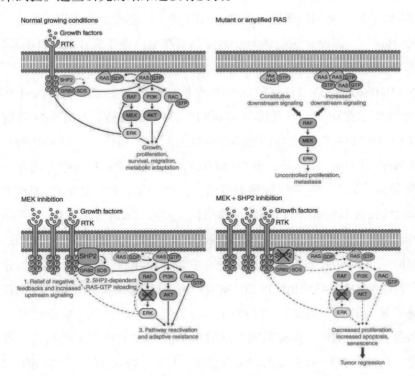

图 5.8　MEK 和 SHP$_2$ 抑制剂的组合是治疗 RAS 驱动的癌症的一种新的治疗方法
　　此图片引自参考文献[146]。

在正常条件下，RTK参与招募RAS-GEF SOS，该程序促进了RAS的GDP对GTP的交换，而该过程对SHP_2的依赖性较低。在具有致癌性*RAS*突变或野生型*RAS*扩增的肿瘤中，RAF-MEK-ERK途径增强。抑制MEK会释放下游负反馈，从而导致RTK活性增强，依赖SHP_2的RAS-GTP负荷增加以及下游信号的重新激活。 MEK和SHP_2的共抑制作用消除了MEK抑制剂诱导的RAS-GTP负荷，并减少了RAS下游的信号传导。

到目前为止所描述的有效的共价$KRAS^{G12C}$抑制剂仅结合与GDP结合的$KRAS^{[106-108]}$，虽然密码子12和13的突变降低了与GDP结合的KRas的比例，但最近的生化分析显示[109]，$KRAS^{G12C}$在*KRAS*突变体中表现出最高的固有GTP水解率和最高的核苷酸交换率。此外，$KRAS^{G12C}$的核苷酸结合状态可以通过用RTK抑制剂对上游信号进行药理学调节来向GDP结合状态转变，RTK抑制剂可以增加$KRAS^{G12C}$抑制剂的活性。同样，SHP_2是一种磷酸酶，能将RTK信号正向转导到KRas[110]。因此，我们认为SHP_2抑制剂在由依赖于核苷酸循环的*KRAS*突变驱动的癌症中是有效的。

PCC0208023也是一种有效的SHP_2变构抑制剂，主要抑制体内SHP_2酶和*KRAS*突变型结直肠癌，以及体外抑制KRas/MAPK途径。与变构抑制模式一致，PCC0208023可以非竞争性地抑制全长SHP_2酶的活性，但对SHP_2的自由催化结构域缺乏活性。在体外，PCC0208023通过抑制KRas/ERK信号通路，抑制*KRAS*突变驱动的人结直肠癌细胞的增殖。重要的是，PCC0208023表现出良好抗*KRAS*驱动的LS180和HCT116异种移植模型对裸鼠KI67和p-ERK水平降低的NTI肿瘤疗效[106]，增加了肿瘤中Caspase-3的切割表达，并且PCC0208023在给药后24h内，LS180肿瘤维持较高水平，主要分布在肠、肺两个部位。分子对接研究表明与RMC-4550相比PCC0208023具有较高的亲和力，SHP_2变构口袋中的关键残基为023（图5.9）。PCC0208023值得进一步优化，以确定额外的低毒性和强效用的SHP_2变构抑制剂与新的用于治疗*KRAS*突变阳性结直肠癌患者的病变。此外，在*KRAS*突变的CRC细胞中，PCC0208023在体外抑制细胞增殖方面比RMC-4550有效。分子对接试验表明，PCC0208023胺基与受体极性相互作用有关，且比RMC-4550受影响更多，这可能是PCC0208023在SHP_2全长酶和

*KRAS*突变CRC细胞中比RMC-4550具有更好的抑制活性的原因。

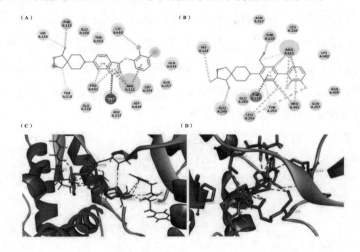

图 5.9   PCC0208023 和 RMC-4550 与 SHP$_2$ 蛋白的分子对接

（A）—PCC0208023的二维（2D）对接结构；（B）—2D对接RMC-4550的构象；（C）—具有SHP$_2$（PDB代码：5EHR）的PCC0208023的对接模式；（D）—PCC0208023和RMC-4550的代表性分子重叠。关键残基用灰色表示，氢键用绿色虚线表示。此图片引用自参考文献[110]。

总之，已经证明PCC0208023是一种有效的变构抑制剂，通过抑制SHP$_2$/RAS/在体外和体内抑制*KRAS*突变型结直肠癌的生长ERK信号通路。进一步优化PCC0208023，以确定更低毒性和更强的SHP$_2$变构抑制剂与新的支架治疗*KRAS*突变阳性CRC是有必要的。

5.2.1.4　Sos 抑制剂

核苷酸交换循环抑制剂Sos抑制剂为最初全球环境基金针对RAS活性发现的一个小分子[111]，它与Switch-Ⅰ和Switch-Ⅱ之间的KRAS结合，从而抑制Sos结合和Sos介导的核苷酸交换。紧接着研究人员试图抑制Sos1-RAS相互作用而尝试使用了一种设计成模仿正交Sos螺旋的分子。虽然该化合物与Sos1结合有纳米摩尔亲和力，遗憾的是，其细胞活性较低[112]。因此该领域把焦点转移到了试图寻找Sos1的小分子抑制剂上，并成功锁定小分子抑制剂BAY-293，该抑制剂通常结合Sos的CDC$_{25}$结构域和RAS-Sos1-RAS三元复合物中与RAS上的Switch-Ⅱ相邻的区域，实验结果提示BAY-293与这个位点的结合可以激活或抑制Sos1-RAS相互作用[113]，且对野生型*KRAS*细胞的增殖抑制作用较强（图5.10）。值得注意的是，BAY-293和*KRAS*^{G12C}共价抑制剂ARS-853在*KRAS*^{G12C}细胞模型中显示出协同的生长抑制效应。这一观察表明，Sos1抑制剂可以与与GDP状态结合的*KRAS*^{G12C}抑制剂联合使用。

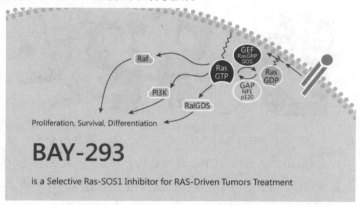

图 5.10　BAY-293 有效破坏了 *KRAS* 及其交换因子 Sos1 之间的相互作用 [113]

此图片引自https://www.cancer-research-network.com/cancer/bay-293-is-a-selective-kras-sos1-inhibitor-for-ras-driven-tumors-treatment/2019-08-31/

5.3　联合途径抑制

最新发表在*Nature*上的一项研究中，来自Memorial Sloan Kettering癌症中心的Piro Lito博士团队揭示了为何*KRAS*^{G12C}抑制剂只能发挥有限的疗效[114]，并且发现了一种克服这类治疗局限性的联合疗法。Lito博士等还发现，癌细胞对*KRAS*^{G12C}抑制剂的这种适应性响应可通过添加第二种药物——AURKA（Aurora Kinase A）抑制剂Alisertib来阻断。Alisertib可帮助保持新产生的*KRAS*^{G12C}蛋白处于可被*KRAS*^{G12C}抑制剂作用的状态。与*KRAS*^{G12C}抑制剂单药治疗相比，AURKA和*KRAS*^{G12C}联合抑制产生了协同的抗增殖作用，导致了更强的抗肿瘤效应[145]。

5.3.1　RAS-效应相互作用抑制剂

虽然针对突变特异性状态对于$KRAS^{G12C}$共价抑制剂是有效的，但要为每个突变的RAS蛋白寻找有效的治疗方法将是困难的。直接靶向所有RAS蛋白（$KRAS$4A、$KRAS$4B、$NRAS$和$HRAS$）上的保守配体结合位点可以提供一种跨越突变和肿瘤类型抑制RAS的单一治疗途径。Welsch等人提出了第一种化合物3144可以在Switch-Ⅰ中结合保守残基Asp38，并阻断RAS与效应器的结合[115]（图5.11）。化合物3144在体外结合野生型$KRAS$、$NRAS$和$HRAS$，在体内抑制$KRAS^{G13D}$肿瘤的生长，但有报告指出，该化合物依然存在不可避免的毒性和靶外活性。事实上，PAN-RAS抑制剂存在很明显的弊端，并且目前我们认为，理论上来说根本不可能取得实质性的成功，因为RAS在正常的细胞信号传递中是必不可少的。所有三种RAS亚型的缺失都会导致小鼠模型中的胚胎死亡[115]。

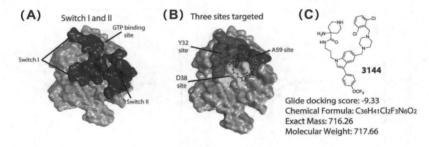

图5.11　RAS蛋白抑制剂3144的设计

（A）—$KRAS^{G12D}$（PDB：4DSN），其中开关Ⅰ区域显示为绿色，而开关Ⅱ区域显示为紫色；（B）—当有3144配体对接时，被靶向的$KRAS^{G12D}$上的三个位点的位置（黄色的D38位点，蓝色的A59位点，红色的Y32位点）；（C）—小分子3144的结构，对接分数，化学式，质量和分子量。此图片引自参考文献[143]。

早期还有研究提出另一种RAS结合小分子DCAⅠ能够轻微抑制Sos1介导的RAS上的核苷酸交换[116]（图5.12）。KRas的结晶表明，DCAⅠ在α2螺旋和核心折叠-Sheetβ1-β3（这里称为DCAⅠ口袋）之间结合了一个口袋，阻止了RAS和Sos1间的相互作用。结合在DCAⅠ口袋中的小分子阻止Sos1介导的鸟嘌呤交换，因此RAS蛋白不能采用GTP结合的活性状态，使这个口袋成为理想的药物靶点。

第三种化合物BI-2852也与DCA I 口袋结合，减少了Sos1介导的交换，从而减少了下游激酶ERK和AKT46的磷酸化，作为PAN-RAS抑制剂发挥作用[116]；DCA I 口袋存在于野生型*RAS*蛋白中，因此这些化合物不是突变选择性抑制剂。需要进一步的研究来优化突变选择性的参数，因为广泛的抑制RAS可能会带来毒性问题。

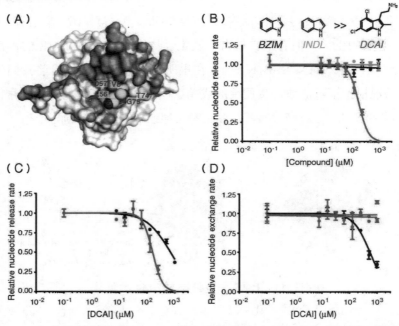

图 5.12　DCA I 特异性抑制 SOScat 催化的核苷酸从 *KRAS* 和 *KRAS*m 释放和交换
（A）—使用HRas-Sos1共晶结构计算Ras / SOS接触表面；（B）—在DCA I（红色）、BZIM（黑色）或INDL（灰色）存在下，用125 nM SOScat一式两份进行SOScat催化的核苷酸释放测定，该图显示了相对于DMSO对照组的速率；（C）—针对野生型 *KRAS*（黑色）和突变体 *KRAS*m（红色）进行SOScat催化的核苷酸释放测定，此处使用了更高的500 nM SOScat浓度来提供 *KRAS*m和 *KRAS*的最佳分析窗口；（D）—在DCA I 存在下，与KRasGDP / SOScat（黑色），RhoAGDP / Dbs（青色）或Cdc42GDP / Dbs（品红色）进行SOScat催化的核苷酸交换反应。此图片引自参考文献[116]。

5.3.2 曲美替尼（Trametinib）联合羟氯喹曲美替尼单药

用于抑制KRas下游的MEK，很容易会在短时间内产生耐药。Trametinib会增加肿瘤细胞的自噬作用[144]，需要加上自噬抑制剂羟氯喹，来加强Trametinib的作用。甲苯达唑有抑制MEK的作用，有加强曲美替尼的作用。

Trametinib与FGFR$_1$抑制剂的联合：通过Trametinib和FGFR$_1$基因抑制剂的联合应用，可以增强FGFR$_1$途径中FGFR受体和配体的活化，抵消Trametinib治疗造成的pFRS2、pERK和pAKT蛋白的增加，协同增强肿瘤细胞死亡。但此作用只针对*KRAS*突变的肺癌和胰腺癌疗效确切，对*KRAS*野生型肺癌和*KRAS*突变的结肠癌细胞则无疗效。

Trametinib与PI3K信号通路抑制剂的联合：*KRAS*能同时激活BRAF与PI3K这两条信号通路，因此单独抑制MEK并不能取得理想的效果，所以需要在抑制MEK的同时，联合抑制PI3K信号通路，比如使用mTOR抑制剂，或者PI3K的抑制剂，或者AKT的抑制剂（MK2206），再或者IGF-1R的抑制剂（OSI-906），也就是说在抑制MEK的同时，在每一个环节中相应地阻断PI3K信号通路，则可能缓解MEK抑制剂的耐药性问题。同时抑制PI3K和MAPK信号通路的临床Ⅰ期试验表明，同时使用两个信号通路的抑制剂，肠癌患者的肿瘤缩小范围在2%～64%之间，呈现出较好的疗效。

5.3.3 MRTX849 联合抑制

在突变癌症的背景下，RTK信号的激活被预测通过增强GTPase活性的外在调节和启动KRas非依赖性ERK和mTOR/S6通路激活来限制MRTX849的治疗反应。因此，HER家族和SHP$_2$抑制分别被用来阻断*KRAS*突变细胞中关键的RTK家族或阻断下游的集体RTK信号。由于MRTX849只与GDP-KRas^{G12C}结合，HER家族和SHP$_2$抑制剂均能增强MRTX849对*KRAS*^{G12C}的修饰，显著提高抗肿瘤活性。这一观察结果与激活的RTK在SHP$_2$参与介导Sos1依赖的RAS GTP负载和降低RAS间隙活性中的假定作用是一致的，RAS激活状态增强可以显著抑制这两种效应[117]。

阿法替尼（Afatinib）抑制EGFR（ErbB1），HER2（ErbB2）和HER4（ErbB4）受体。Afatinib与MRTX849联合应用对ERK/RSK和AKT-mTOR/S6信号通路均有明显抑制作用；SHP$_2$抑制剂与MRTX849联合应用对ERK/RSK信号转导也有明显影响，对mTOR/S6信号转导影响相对较小。虽然Afatinib可以更有效地解决mTOR/S6旁路信号，但我们认为SHP$_2$抑制对于对抗HER家族以外的其他RTK，如FGFRs或MET，是一种更为有效的组合策略，这些可能对KRas依赖产生有利的影响。除此之外，mTOR抑制剂与MRTX849联合使用也被评估，研究数据提示可能对于解决由RTK激活或STK$_{11}$突变介导的旁路信号产生积极作用。这两种信号通路中的每一种都独立于KRas激活mTOR/S6信号通路。

正向研究数据表明，MRTX849与Vistusertib联合使用，与任何一种药物相比，体内抗肿瘤活性都有显著提高，而这些结果与STK$_{11}$突变状态无关。与Vistusertib的作用机制一致，单用Vistusertib可全面抑制AKT-mTOR/S6信号转导，与MRTX849联合应用可几乎完全抑制pS6$^{S235/36}$和$^{S240/44}$。此外，vistusertib对ERK的反馈再激活也因联合作用而减轻[118-120]。因此，我们认为这些都是支持与MRTX849联合抑制ERK信号的一个关键机制。

值得注意的是，所有三种组合策略都在更全面地抑制ERK和S6活性的KRas依赖信号上比较相似。此外，虽然AKT-mTOR/S6的抑制与MRTX849的模型反应无关（可能是由于肿瘤的异质性），但观察到mTOR和RPS6都在药物锚定的CRISPR筛查中消失，有效的联合策略更全面地阻断了这一途径，这表明它在最大化抑制*KRAS*突变癌症的治疗反应方面可能具有重要意义。由于细胞周期调节器的遗传改变导致的细胞周期失调，确定了可能改变MRTX849治疗反应的额外因素。此外，在CRISPR筛查中，CDKN2A、RB1、CDK4和CDK6都被鉴定为影响细胞适合性的基因靶点。包括CDKN2A纯合缺失或CDK4或CCND1扩增在内的遗传改变占*KRAS*突变的NSCLC的20%[121]。体内联合应用MRTX849和Palbociclib的研究表明，在NSCLC模型中，与单药相比，MRTX849和Palbociclib对Rb和E$_2$F家族靶基因的抑制作用更全面，抗肿瘤活性更强。此外，这些研究表明，联合使用能更有效地抑制S6（S235/236）磷酸化，从而在细胞周期阻滞和蛋白质翻译途径之间建立了以前不为人知的联系。这种联合在

CDKN2A缺失的模型中特别有效，表明这种联合策略可能在以细胞周期调节与KRas解耦患者受益为主。

有研究在单药MRTX849治疗未显示持久回归的模型中，选择5个模型（KYSE410、SW1573、H2122、H2030、LU6405）进行合理组合研究[121]，其中至少有一个组合的抗肿瘤效果显著改善，在所有评价的5个模型中，肿瘤消退率平均达到50%。这些结果表明，基本上所有$KRAS^{G12C}$突变的癌症都可以从直接的$KRAS$抑制剂治疗中获得临床益处，无论是单独治疗还是联合治疗。此外，针对MARK信号节点的以通路为中心的联合方案可能针对基因定义的患者亚群有利。总之研究结果提示，$KRAS^{G12C}$/STK11突变的NSCLC可以通过$KRAS^{G12C}$抑制剂与RTK或mTOR抑制剂联合使用来解决，而$KRAS^{G12C}$/CDKN2A突变的NSCLC可以通过联合CDK4/6抑制剂更有效地解决[122-123]。

6 　总结与展望

　　我们认为$KRAS^{G12C}$等位基因特异性抑制剂有可能改变$KRAS$驱动的肿瘤的治疗格局。这些抑制剂有望成为FDA批准的第一种治疗$KRAS$突变肿瘤的药物，并将用于治疗由突变$KRAS$驱动的PDAC、CRC和LUAD等难以治愈的实体瘤。尽管这些抑制剂的发展令人难以置信地兴奋，但新的挑战和问题将会出现。

　　继续开发针对其他等位基因的特异性抑制剂是首要任务，如$KRAS^{G12D}$和$KRAS^{G12V}$，这些等位基因是最常见的$KRAS$变异，因此与最大的患者群体相关。最终，可以针对所有突变的$KRAS$等位基因开发特异性抑制剂，从而提供一种个性化的药物治疗方法。靶向突变的$KRAS$蛋白是治疗$KRAS$突变肿瘤的最佳方法。然而，等位基因特异性抑制剂作为单一疗法的疗效可能有限，最大化的抗肿瘤效果需要与其他抑制剂联合使用。

　　确定哪种组合策略在患者身上效果最好十分具有挑战性。首先，$KRAS$的每一种变异都有不同的生化特性，这些特性将决定对所讨论的许多治疗方法的反应。我们认为SHP_2和$KRAS^{G12C}$抑制剂联合使用将是一种有效的治疗策略。了解特定突变型RAS密码子的要求和抑制剂对这些等位基因的反应，对于开发战略性联合疗法是必要的。第二，正如本综述中$KRAS$突变的临床意义部分所讨论的，肿瘤类型可以显著影响应答率。$KRAS$突变导致的CRC和PDAC对MAPK抑制剂或免疫点阻断的反应最小。AMG 510试验的早期数据显示，结直肠癌比LUAD更难治，这表明结直肠癌将需要联合治疗。大肠癌的治疗尤其具有挑战性。然而，用曲美替尼、恩可拉非尼和西妥昔单抗三联用药在$BRAF^{V600E}$转移性大肠癌中观察到了有希望的抗肿瘤效果，这表明KRAS突变的大肠癌将需要一种积极的联合策略才能达到应答[124]。第三，目前为止，联合治疗一直有毒性大、安全保障小等弊端。仅AMG 510观察到通过减少剂量对限制毒性有一定的成效，突变特异性治疗应该具有有限的非靶点效应。等位基因特异性抑制剂（低毒）可以与其他毒性更大的抑制剂联合使用，才能尽可能地避免与PI3K和MEK抑制剂联合使用时观察到的两种有毒化合物组合的问题。

随着KRAS驱动的肿瘤的治疗变得更加个性化，另一个亟待解决的挑战在于评估对等位基因特异性抑制的潜在耐药机制。肿瘤的异质性可以提供内在的耐药机制。例如，一个肿瘤可能含有95%的$KRAS^{G12C}$和0.1%的$KRAS^{G12V}$细胞。在使用等位基因特异性的$KRAS^{G12C}$抑制剂治疗后，肿瘤会消退，但如果选择$KRAS^{G12V}$细胞，肿瘤会复发[125]。肿瘤的异质性也可能导致出现内在耐药的问题，因为亚群细胞对$KRAS^{G12C}$抑制具有耐药性。临床目前现有的模型还没有考虑到肿瘤的异质性。目前，几乎没有证据表明在使用$KRAS^{G12C}$等位基因特异性抑制剂治疗时会出现哪些类型的从头突变[125]。

已经描述的EGFR和BRAF-V600抑制剂的耐药机制可能有助于我们在临床上看到等位基因特异性$KRAS^{G12C}$抑制剂的从头突变。正如在共价EGFR抑制剂中观察到的那样，半胱氨酸突变是一种预期的耐药机制[126]；然而，在$KRAS^{G12C}$的情况下，半胱氨酸突变是致癌活性所必需的，因此这不太可能在临床上实现。基因扩增为抵抗BRAF-V600抑制剂的首要分子机制[127-128]，并在EGFR抑制剂的背景下观察到MET扩增[129]。在这种情况下，EGFR或其他上游EGFR家族成员的扩增可能导致细胞内GTP结合的RAS水平升高，从而对$KRAS^{G12C}$抑制剂产生耐药性，因为这些分子与GDP结合。此外，RAS扩增，无论是HRAS还是NRAS，或者KRAS本身的扩增都可能导致RAS二聚化和GTP结合的RAS水平升高，从而对$KRAS^{G12C}$抑制剂产生抗性。在BRAF突变的肿瘤中，大多数获得性耐药机制都需要重新激活MAPK通路，除了上述机制外，这还可以通过NRAS和MEK1/2的突变来实现[130-131]。因此，MAPK通路的重新激活提供了许多有待被发现的抵抗等位基因特异性抑制剂的靶点，并且可以通过改变上游信号（通过EGFR突变或扩增，或RAS扩增）或下游机制，如RAF或MEK突变来实现。

像分泌前肝素可以结合EGF样生长因子一样，EGFR可以通过自分泌和/或旁分泌机制重新被激活[125]。然而，目前还不清楚这些机制是否会在RAS突变或肿瘤类型中与预测假想保持一致。

综上所述，靶向KRAS还存在着许多未知的问题亟待解决，同时也意味着靶向治疗还存在着无限的可能性。因此，我们提出了一种崭新的思路：靶向突变型KRAS核酸蛋白复合物的设计，CRISPR-Cas9 系统是目前基因编辑领域最受欢迎的新技术，未来它将改变人们治疗疾病的方式。已开发的常用CRISPR-Cas9系统有两部分组成：引导RNA和核酸内切酶（Cas9）。gRNA可以引导Cas9蛋白结合到基因组靶基因处，行使核酸内切酶功能切割靶基因双链DNA，利用细胞的非同源末端连接或同源重组修复机制对断裂的DNA进行插入缺失、修复或者替换，实现高效基因编辑[132]。Cas9的核酸内切酶活性取决于RuvC和HNH这两个结构域，分别负责切割DNA的两条链[133]。当这两个结构域同时被人工点突变（D10A和H840A）后，会造成Cas9丧失核酸内切酶活性成为deadCas9（dCas9），但dCas9仍然可以在gRNA的引导下与基因组中特定的DNA序列相结合。当dCas9蛋白与转录激活因子或阻遏蛋白融合时，可以将其工程化为转录调控因子，调节基因的表达[134]。

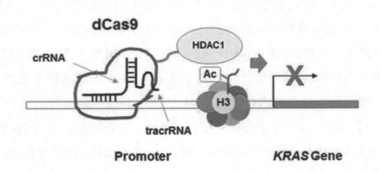

图 6.1　通过表观基因组编辑设计用于 K-Ras 沉默的 dCas9-HDAC1 融合蛋白
crRNA将dCas9-HDAC1融合蛋白引导至KRAS启动子。启动子处的组蛋白去乙酰化抑制癌细胞中突变K-Ras表达。

基于以上原理，我们针对含有突变型 *KRAS* 的肿瘤细胞设计了一种新颖的核酸蛋白复合物（dCas9–HDAC1–sgRNA$_{KRAS}$），目标是在不改变基因组 DNA 遗传信息的前提下，通过表观基因组编辑抑制 KRas 突变体蛋白的表达。此核酸蛋白复合物主要由以下两部分组成：①dCas9 和组蛋白去乙酰基酶1（HDAC1）构成的融合蛋白——dCas9–HDAC1；②包含有与 *KRAS* 启动子区结合的 crRNA 序列和 tracrRNA 序列的 sgRNA$_{KRAS}$。我们的策略是：在 sgRNA$_{KRAS}$ 的引导下，融合蛋白 dCas9–HDAC1 与 *KRAS* 启动子区相结合，而组蛋白去乙酰基化是表观遗传领域抑制基因表达的一个标志[135]，HDAC1 可以使 *KRAS* 启动子区核心组蛋白 N 端部分的赖氨酸残基去乙酰基化后，与带负电荷的 DNA 结合变得紧密，染色质致密卷曲，从而达到抑制 *KRAS* 的转录表达的目的（图6.1）。希望我们的思路可以为 *KRAS* 靶向抑制的研究带来新策略和实验依据，让"不可成药"成为过去式。

参考文献

[1] 陈薄羲. Kras 基因性质与结构分析 [J]. 当代化工研究，2019（02）：184-186.

[2] ALEMAYEHU A G，BARRY G B，MCCAMMON J A. Mapping the nucleotide and isoform-dependent structural and dynamical features of Ras proteins[J]. Structure，2008，16（6）：885-896.

[3] ALEMAYEHU A G，HANZAL B M，ABANKWA D，et al. Structure and dynamics of the full-length lipid-modified H-Ras protein in a 1，2-dimyristoylglycero-3-phosphocholine bilayer[J]. Journal of medicinal chemistry，2007，50（4）：674-684.

[4] ABANKWA D，GORFE A A，HANCOCK J F. Mechanisms of Ras membrane organization and signaling：Ras on a rocker[J]. Cell Cycle，2008，7（17）：2667-2673.

[5] JOHN J，SCHLICHTING I，SCHILTZ E，et al. C-terminal truncation of p21H preserves crucial kinetic and structural properties[J]. Journal of Biological Chemistry，1989，264（22）：13086.

[6] AHMADIAN M R，WIESMULLER L，LAUTWEIN A，et al. Structural differences in the minimal catalytic domains of the GTPase-activating proteins p120GAP and neurofibromin[J]. Journal of biological chemistry，1996，271（27）：16409-16415.

[7] BUHRMAN G，HOLZAPFEL G，FETICS S，et al. Allosteric modulation of Ras positions Q61 for a direct role in catalysis[J]. Proceedings of the National Academy of Sciences of the United States of America，2010，107（11）：4931-4936.

[8] PRIOR I A，HOOD F E，HARTLEY J L. The frequency of Ras mutations in cancer[J]. Cancer Research，2020，80（14）：3682.

[9] HOBBS G A，DER C J，ROSSMAN K L. RAS isoforms and mutations in cancer at a glance[J]. Journal of cell science，2016：1287.

[10] PRIOR I A, LEWIS P D, MATTOS C. A comprehensive survey of Ras mutations in cancer[J]. Cancer Research, 2012, 72（10）: 2457-2467.

[11] LAUDE A J, PRIOR I A. Palmitoylation and localisation of RAS isoforms are modulated by the hypervariable linker domain[J]. Journal of cell science, 2008, 121（4）: 421.

[12] TSAI F D, LOPES M S, ZHOU M, et al. K-Ras4A splice variant is widely expressed in cancer and uses a hybrid membrane-targeting motif[J]. Proceedings of the national academy of sciences of the United States of America, 2015, 112（3）: 779-784.

[13] MCGRATH J P, CAPON D J, SMITH D H, et al. Structure and organization of the human K-ras proto-oncogene and a related processed pseudogene[J]. Nature, 1983, 304（5926）.

[14] PELLS S, DIVJAK M, ROMANOWSKI P, et al. Developmentally-regulated expression of murine K-ras isoforms. [J]. Oncogene, 1997, 15（15）: 1781-1786.

[15] PLOWMAN S J, BERRY R L, BADER S A, et al. K-ras 4A and 4B are co-expressed widely in human tissues, and their ratio is altered in sporadic colorectal cancer[J]. Journal of experimental & Clinical cancer research Cr, 2006, 25（2）: 259-267.

[16] CHEN W C, MINH D T, PETER M K, et al. Regulation of KRAS4A/B splicing in cancer stem cells by the RBM39 splicing complex[J]. Preprint at bioRxiv, 2019.

[17] CHERFILS J, ZEGHOUF M. Regulation of small GTPases by GEFs, GAPs, and GDIs[J]. Physiological reviews, 2013, 93（1）: 269-309.

[18] ZARBL H, SUKUMAR S, ARTHUR A V, et al. Direct mutagenesis of Ha-ras-1 oncogenes by N-nitroso-N-methylurea during initiation of mammary carcinogenesis in rats[J]. Nature, 1985, 315（6018）: 382-385.

[19] BARBACID M. Ras Oncogenes: their role in neoplasia[J]. European journal of clinical investigation, 1990, 20（3）: 225-235.

[20] DONNA M, MUZNY, MATTHEW N, et al. Comprehensive molecular characterization of human colon and rectal cancer. [J]. Nature, 2012, 487（7407）: 330-337.

[21] ERIC A, COLLISSON J D, CAMPBELL A N, et al. Comprehensive molecular profiling of lung adenocarcinoma[J]. Nature, 2014, 511（7511）: 543-550.

[22] RAPHAEL B J, HRUBAN R H, AGUIRRE A J, et al. Integrated genomic characterization of pancreatic ductal adenocarcinoma[J]. Cancer Cell, 2017, 32（2）: 185-203.

[23] FRIEDLAENDER A, DRILON A, WEISS G J, et al. KRAS as a druggable target in NSCLC: Rising like a phoenix after decades of development failures[J]. Cancer Treatment

Reviews, 2020, 85: 101978.

[24] National Comprehensive Cancer Network （NCCN）. NCCN clinical practice guidelines in oncology[J]. Uterine Neoplasms, 2011, 1.

[25] JOHNSON C W, LIN Y J, REID D. Isoform-specific destabilization of the active site reveals a molecular mechanism of intrinsic activation of KRas G13D[J]. Cell Reports, 2019, 28（6）: 1538-1550.

[26] MOORE M J, GOLDSTEIN D, HAMM J, et al. Erlotinib plus gemcitabine compared with gemcitabine alone in patients with advanced pancreatic cancer: a phase III trial of the National Cancer Institute of Canada Clinical Trials Group[J]. Journal of clinical oncology: official journal of the American Society of Clinical Oncology, 2007, 25（15）: 1960-1966.

[27] AMODIO V, YAEGER R, ARCELLA P, et al. EGFR blockade reverts resistance to KRAS G12C inhibition in colorectal cancer[J]. Cancer Discovery, 2020, 10（8）: CD-20-0187.

[28] LINARDOU H. Assessment of somatic k-RAS mutations as a mechanism associated with resistance to EGFR-targeted agents: a systematic review and meta-analysis of studies in advanced non-small-cell lung cancer and metastatic colorectal cancer[J]. Lancet Oncol, 2008, 9（10）: 962-972.

[29] MAO C, QIU L X, LIAO R Y, et al. KRAS mutations and resistance to EGFR-TKIs treatment in patients with non-small cell lung cancer: A meta-analysis of 22 studies[J]. Lung Cancer, 2010, 69（3）: 272-278.

[30] PAO W. EGF receptor gene mutations are common in lung cancers from "never smokers" and are associated with sensitivity of tumors to gefitinib and erlotinib[J]. Proc Natl Acad Sci USA, 2004, 101（36）: 13306-13311.

[31] KOBAYASHI S, BOGGON T J, DAYARAM T, et al. EGFR mutation and resistance of non-small-cell lung cancer to gefitinib[J]. The New England Jouranl of Medcine, 2005, 352（8）: 786-792.

[32] COLLINS M A, BEDNAR F, ZHANG Y, et al. Oncogenic Kras is required for both the initiation and maintenance of pancreatic cancer in mice[J]. The Journal of clinical investigation, 2012, 122（2）: 639-653.

[33] SHANKAR S, PITCHIAYA S, MALIK R, et al. KRAS engages AGO2 to enhance cellular transformation[J]. Cell Reports, 2016, 14（6）: 1448-1461.

[34] SHIPMAN L. Anticancer drugs: Putting the brakes on KRAS-G12C nucleotide cycling[J].

Nature Reviews Drug Discovery, 2016, 15（3）: 159-159.

[35] ATHULURI D S K, CARPIO V D, DUTTA K, et al. A small molecule RAS-mimetic disrupts RAS association with effector proteins to block signaling[J]. Cell, 2016, 165（3）: 643-655.

[36] BIVONA T G, QUATELA S E, BODEMANN B O, et al. PKC regulates a farnesyl-electrostatic switch on K-Ras that promotes its association with Bcl-X l on mitochondria and induces apoptosis[J]. Molecular Cell, 2006, 21（4）: 481-493.

[37] PADANAD M, KONSTANTINIDOU G, VENKATESWARAN N, et al. Fatty acid oxidation mediated by Acyl-CoA synthetase long chain 3 is required for mutant KRAS lung tumorigenesis[J]. Cell Reports, 2016, 16（6）: 1614-1628.

[38] WANG J, HU K, GUO J, et al. Suppression of KRas-mutant cancer through the combined inhibition of KRAS with PLK1 and ROCK[J]. Nature Communications, 2016, 7: 11363.

[39] FENG H, ZHANG Y, BOS P H, et al. K-RasG12D has a potential allosteric small molecule binding site[J]. Biochemistry, 2019, 58（21）.

[40] HUNTER J C, MANANDHAR A, CARRASCO M A, et al. Biochemical and structural analysis of common cancer-associated KRAS mutations [J]. Molecular Cancer Research Mcr, 2015, 13（9）: 1325-1335.

[41] CANON J, REX K, SAIKI A Y, et al. The clinical KRAS（G12C）inhibitor AMG 510 drives anti-tumour immunity[J]. Nature, 2019, 575（7781）: 217-223.

[42] Amgen. Amgen Announces New Clinical Data Evaluating Novel Investigational KRAS（G12C）Inhibitor in Patients with Solid Tumors at ESMO 2019.

[43] TSHERNIAK A, VAZQUEZ F, MONTGOMERY P G, et al. Defining a cancer dependency map[J]. Cell, 2017, 170（3）: 564-576.

[44] CHRISTENSEN J G, HALLIN J, ENGSTROM L D, et al. The KRASG12C inhibitor MRTX849 provides insight toward therapeutic susceptibility of KRAS-mutant cancers in mouse models and patients[J]. Cancer Discovery, 2019, 10（1）: CD-19-1167.

[45] JANES M R, ZHANG J, LI L S, et al. Targeting KRAS mutant cancers with a covalent G12C-Specific inhibitor-science direct[J]. Cell, 2018, 172（3）: 578-589.

[46] MCDONALD E R, ANTOINE D W, MICHAEL R, et al. Project drive: A compendium of cancer dependencies and synthetic lethal relationships uncovered by large-scale, deep RNAi screening[J]. Cell, 2017, 170（3）: 577-592.

[47] LITO P，PRATILAS C A，JOSEPH E W，et al. Relief of profound feedback inhibition of mitogenic signaling by RAF inhibitors attenuates their activity in BRAFV600E melanomas[J]. Cancer Cell，2012，22（5）：668-682.

[48] HANAFUSA H，TORII S，T YASUNAGA，et al. Sprouty1 and Sprouty2 provide a control mechanism for the Ras/MAPK signalling pathway[J]. Nature cell biology，2002，4（11）：850-858.

[49] CHRISTENSEN J G，HALLIN J，ENGSTROM L D，et al. The KRASG12C inhibitor MRTX849 provides insight toward therapeutic susceptibility of KRAS-mutant cancers in mouse models and patients[J]. Cancer Discovery，2019，10（1）：54-71.

[50] SANTANA C N，CHANDHOKE A S，YU Q，et al. Defining and targeting adaptations to oncogenic KRAS G12C inhibition using quantitative temporal proteomics[J]. Cell Reports，2020，30（13）：4584-4599.

[51] CARTER C A. Selumetinib with and without erlotinib in KRAS mutant and KRAS wild-type advanced nonsmall-cell lung cancer[J]. Ann. Oncol，2016，27（4）：693-699.

[52] JANNE P，VAN D H M，BARLESI F，et al. Selumetinib plus docetaxel compared with docetaxel alone and progression-free survival in patients with KRAS-mutant advanced non - small cell lung cancer：the select-1 randomized clinical trial[J]. Jama，2017，317（18）：1844-1853.

[53] HELLMANN M D，KIM T W，LEE C B，et al. Phase Ib study of atezolizumab combined with cobimetinib in patients with solid tumors[J]. Annals of Oncology，2019，30（7）：1134-1142.

[54] FRIDAY B B，YU C，DY G K，et al. BRAF V600E disrupts AZD6244-induced abrogation of negative feedback pathways between extracellular signal-regulated kinase and Raf proteins[J]. Cancer Research，2008，68（15）：6145-6153.

[55] HATZIVASSILIOU G. Mechanism of MEK inhibition determines efficacy in mutant KRAS-versus BRAF-driven cancers[J]. Nature，2013，501（7466）：232-236.

[56] LITO P. Disruption of CRAF-mediated MEK activation is required for effective MEK inhibition in KRAS mutant tumors[J]. Cancer Cell，2014，25（50）：697-710.

[57] BLUMENSCHEIN G R. A randomized phase II study of the MEK1/MEK2 inhibitor trametinib （GSK1120212）compared with docetaxel in KRAS-mutant advanced non-small-cell lung cancer（NSCLC）[J]. Annals of Oncology Official Journal of the European Society for Medical

Oncology, 2015, 26（5）.

[58] YEN I, SHANAHAN F, MERCHANT M, et al. Pharmacological induction of RAS-GTP confers RAF inhibitor sensitivity in KRAS mutant tumors[J]. Cancer Cell, 2018, 34（4）: 611-625.

[59] MORRIS E J, JHA S, RESTAINO C R, et al. Discovery of a novel ERK inhibitor with activity in models of acquired resistance to BRAF and MEK inhibitors[J]. Cancer discovery, 2013, 3（7）: 742-750.

[60] HATZIVASSILIOU G, LIU B, O"BRIEN C, et al. ERK inhibition overcomes acquired resistance to MEK inhibitors[J]. Molecular Cancer Therapeutics, 2012, 11（5）: 1143.

[61] CHAIKUAD A, ELIANA M C T, ZIMMER J, et al. A unique inhibitor binding site in ERK1/2 is associated with slow binding kinetics[J]. Nature Chemical Biology, 2014, 10（10）: 853.

[62] MOSCHOS S J, SULLIVAN R J, HWU W J, et al. Development of MK-8353, an orally administered ERK1/2 inhibitor, in patients with advanced solid tumors[J]. Jci Insight, 2018, 3（4）.

[63] He Y, Li Y, Qiu Z, et al. Identification and validation of PROM1 and CRTC2 mutations in lung cancer patients[J]. Molecular Cancer, 2014, 13（1）: 19.

[64] BOGA S B, DENG Y Q, ZHU L, et al. MK-8353: Discovery of an orally bioavailable dual mechanism ERK inhibitor for oncology[J]. ACS medicinal chemistry letters, 2018, 9（7）.

[65] MERCHANT M, MOFFAT J, SCHAEFER G, et al. Combined MEK and ERK inhibition overcomes therapy-mediated pathway reactivation in RAS mutant tumors[J]. Plos One, 2018, 13（1）.

[66] WEEKES C, LOCKHART A, LORUSSO P, et al. A Phase Ib study to evaluate the MEK inhibitor cobimetinib in combination with the ERK1/2 inhibitor GDC-0994 in patients with advanced solid tumors[J]. The oncologist, 2020, 25（10）.

[67] VARGA A, SORIA J C, HOLLEBECQUE A, et al. A First-in-human phase I study to evaluate the ERK1/2 inhibitor GDC-0994 in patients with advanced solid tumors[J]. European Journal of Cancer, 2016, 12（69）: S11.

[68] BURROWS F, KESSLER L, CHEN J, et al. Abstract 5168: KO-947, a potent ERK inhibitor with robust preclinical single agent activity in MAPK pathway dysregulated tumors[J]. Cancer Research, 2017, 77（13）: 5168-5168.

[69] BHAGWAT S V, MCMILLEN W T, CAI S, et al. Abstract 4973: Discovery of LY3214996, a selective and novel ERK1/2 inhibitor with potent antitumor activities in cancer models with MAPK pathway alterations[J]. Cancer Research, 2017, 77 (13): 4973-4973.

[70] PANT S, BENDELL J C, SULLIVAN R J, et al. A phase I dose escalation (DE) study of ERK inhibitor, LY3214996, in advanced (adv) cancer (CA) patients (pts) [J]. Journal of Clinical Oncology, 2019, 37 (15): 3001.

[71] XIE Y Y, CAO Z, WONG E W, et al. COP1-DET1-ETS axis regulates ERK transcriptome and sensitivity to MAPK inhibitors[J]. Journal of Clinical Investigation, 2018, 128 (4): 1442-1457.

[72] DOUGHERTY M K, JÜRGEN M, RITT D A, et al. Regulation of Raf-1 by direct feedback phosphorylation[J]. Molecular Cell, 2005, 17 (2): 215-224.

[73] LAKE D, CORRÊA, SONIA A L, MÜLLER JÜRGEN. Negative feedback regulation of the ERK1/2 MAPK pathway[J]. Cellular & Molecular Life Sciences, 2016, 73 (23): 4397-4413.

[74] KIM H J, BAR-SAGI D. Modulation of signalling by Sprouty: a developing story[J]. Nature Reviews Molecular Cell Biology, 2004, 5 (6): 441-450.

[75] KAROULIA Z, WU Y, TAMER A, et al. An integrated model of RAF inhibitor action predicts inhibitor activity against oncogenic BRAF signaling[J]. Cancer Cell, 2016: 485-498.

[76] GEORGIA H, KYUNG S, IVANA Y, et al. RAF inhibitors prime wild-type RAF to activate the MAPK pathway and enhance growth[J]. Nature, 2010, 464 (7287): 431-435.

[77] YEN I, SHANAHAN F, MERCHANT M, et al. Pharmacological induction of RAS-GTP confers RAF inhibitor sensitivity in KRAS mutant tumors[J]. Cancer Cell, 2018, 34 (4): 611-625.

[78] SHENG B P, JAMES R H, MICHAEL D K, et al. Inhibition of RAF isoforms and active dimers by LY3009120 leads to anti-tumor activities in RAS or BRAF mutant cancers[J]. Cancer Cell, 2015, 28 (3): 384-398.

[79] WANG X, KIM J. Conformation-specific effects of Raf kinase inhibitors[J]. Journal of Medicinal Chemistry, 2012, 55 (17): 7332-7341.

[80] KIM T W, LEE J, SHIN S J, et al. Belvarafenib, a novel pan-RAF inhibitor, in solid tumor patients harboring BRAF, KRAS, or NRAS mutations: phase I study[J]. Clin. Oncol, 2019, 37 (15): 3000.

[81] MONACO K A. RAF inhibitor LXH254 effectively inhibits B-and-CRAF, but not ARAF [J]. Cancer Res. , 2019, 79（Suppl. 13）, LB-144.

[82] SULLIVAN R J, HOLLEBECQUE A, FLAHERTY K T, et al. A phase I study of LY3009120, a Pan-RAF inhibitor, in patients with advanced or metastatic cancer[J]. Molecular Cancer Therapeutics, 2020, 19（2）: 460-467.

[83] VANHAESEBROECK B, WELHAM M J, KOTANI K, et al. P110δ, a novel phosphoinositide 3-kinase in leukocytes[J]. Proceedings of the National Academy of Sciences of the United States of America, 1997, 94（9）: 4330-4335.

[84] HIRSCH E, Vladimir L K, Cecilia G, et al. Central role for G protein-coupled phosphoinositide 3-kinase γ in inflammation[J]. Science, 2000, 287（5455）: 1049-1053.

[85] Houslay D M, Anderson K E, Chessa T, et al. Coincident signals from GPCRs and receptor tyrosine kinases are uniquely transduced by PI3Kβ in myeloid cells[J]. Science Signaling, 2016, 9（441）: ra82.

[86] Schmid M, Avraamides C, Dippold H, et al. Receptor tyrosine kinases and TLR/IL1Rs unexpectedly activate myeloid cell PI3Kγ, A single convergent point promoting tumor inflammation and progression[J]. Cancer cell, 2011, 19（6）: 715-727.

[87] BACHMAN K E, ARGANI P, SAMUELS Y, et al. The PIK3CA gene is mutated with high frequency in human breast cancers[J]. Cancer Biology & Therapy, 2004, 3（8）: 772-775.

[88] JING, YEN, CLIFFORD. PTEN, a putative protein tyrosine phosphatase gene mutated in human brain, breast, and prostate cancer[J]. Science, 1997, 275（5308）: 1943-1947.

[89] QIANG W, YAN L S, KAI Z, et al. PIK3CA mutations confer resistance to first-line chemotherapy in colorectal cancer[J]. Cell Death & Disease, 2018, 9（7）: 739.

[90] WEE S, JAGANI Z, XIANG K X, et al. PI3K pathway activation mediates resistance to MEK inhibitors in KRAS mutant cancers. [J]. Cancer Research, 2009, 69（10）: 4286-4293.

[91] ENGELMAN J A, CHEN L, TAN X, et al. Effective use of PI3K and MEK inhibitors to treat mutant Kras G12D and PIK3CA H1047R murine lung cancers[J]. Nature medicine, 2008, 14（12）: 1351-1356.

[92] HOEFLICH K P, MERCHANT M, ORR C, et al. Intermittent administration of MEK inhibitor GDC-0973 plus PI3K inhibitor GDC-0941 triggers robust apoptosis and tumor growth

inhibition[J]. Cancer Research, 2012, 72（1）: 210-219.

[93] ALGAZI A P, ROTOW J, POSCH C, et al. A dual pathway inhibition strategy using BKM120 combined with vemurafenib is poorly tolerated in BRAF V600E/K mutant advanced melanoma[J]. Pigment Cell & Melanoma Research, 2019, 32（1）.

[94] MOLINA A M, HANCOCK D C, SHERIDAN C, et al. Coordinate direct input of both KRAS and IGF1 receptor to activation of PI 3-kinase in KRAS mutant lung cancer[J]. Cancer Discovery, 2013, 3（5）: 548-563.

[95] SHI Z Q, YU D H, PARK M, et al. Molecular mechanism for the Shp-2 tyrosine phosphatase function in promoting growth factor stimulation of erk activity[J]. Molecular & Cellular Biology, 2000, 20（5）: 1526-1536.

[96] RUESS D A, HEYNEN G J, CIECIELSKI K J, et al. Mutant KRAS-driven cancers depend on PTPN11/SHP2 phosphatase[J]. Nature Medicine, 2018, 24（7）: 954-960.

[97] GROSSMANN K S, MARTA ROSÁRIO, BIRCHMEIER C, et al. The tyrosine phosphatase Shp2 in development and cancer. [J]. Advances in Cancer Research, 2010, 106: 53-89.

[98] RAMADAN W S, VAZHAPPILLY C G, SALEH E M, et al. Interplay between epigenetics, expression of estrogen Receptor-α, HER2/ERBB2 and sensitivity of triple negative breast cancer cells to hormonal therapy[J]. Cancers, 2018, 11（1）: 13.

[99] NICHOLS R J, FRANZISKA H, CARLOS S, et al. RAS nucleotide cycling underlies the SHP2 phosphatase dependence of mutant BRAF-, NF1- and RAS-driven cancers[J]. Nature Cell Biology, 2018, 20（9）: 1064-1073.

[100] DANCE M, MONTAGNER A, SALLES J P, et al. The molecular functions of Shp2 in the Ras/Mitogen-activated protein kinase（ERK1/2）pathway[J]. Cellular Signalling, 2008, 20（3）: 453-459.

[101] BENNETT A M, TANG T L, SUGIMOTO S, et al. Protein-tyrosine-phosphatase SHPTP2 couples platelet-derived growth factor receptor beta to Ras[J]. Proceedings of the National Academy of Sciences of the United States of America, 1994, 91（15）: 7335-7339.

[102] Ruess D A, Heynen G J, Ciecielski K J, et al. Mutant KRAS-driven cancers depend on PTPN11/SHP2 phosphatase[J]. Nature Medicine, 2018, 24（7）: 954-960.

[103] Nichols R J, Franziska H, Carlos S, et al. RAS nucleotide cycling underlies the SHP2 phosphatase dependence of mutant BRAF-, NF1- and RAS-driven cancers[J]. Nature Cell Biology, 2018, 20（9）: 1064-1073.

[104] Mirati Therapeutics. Mirati announces clinical collaboration to evaluate MRTX849 in combination with SHP2 inhibitor[J]. Mirati, 2019.

[105] JANES M R, ZHANG J, LI L S, et al. Targeting KRAS mutant cancers with a covalent G12C-specific inhibitor[J]. Cell, 2018, 172（3）: 578-589.

[106] OSTREM J M, PETERS U, SOS M L, et al. K-Ras（G12C）inhibitors allosterically control GTP affinity and effector interactions. [J]. Nature, 2013, 503（7477）: 548-551.

[107] PATRICELLI M P, JANES M R, LI L S, et al. Selective inhibition of oncogenic KRAS output with small molecules targeting the inactive state[J]. Cancer Discovery, 2016, 6（3）: 316-329.

[108] HUNTER J C, MANANDHAR A, CARRASCO M A, et al. Biochemical and structural analysis of common cancer-associated KRAS mutations[J]. Molecular Cancer Research Mcr, 2015, 13（9）: 1325-1335.

[109] CHEN X, ZOU F, HU Z, et al. PCC0208023, a potent SHP2 allosteric inhibitor, imparts an antitumor effect against KRAS mutant colorectal cancer[J]. Toxicology and Applied Pharmacology, 2020, 398: 115019.

[110] SUN Q, JASON. Discovery of small molecules that bind to K-Ras and inhibit Sos-mediated activation[J]. Angewandte Chemie （International ed. in English）, 2012, 51（25）: 6140-6143.

[111] LESHCHINER E S, PARKHITKO A, BIRD G H, et al. Direct inhibition of oncogenic KRAS by hydrocarbon-stapled SOS1 helices[J]. Proceedings of the National Academy of Sciences of the United States of America, 2015, 112（6）: 1761-1766.

[112] HILLIG R C, SAUTIER B, SCHROEDER J, et al. PNAS Plus: Discovery of potent SOS1 inhibitors that block RAS activation via disruption of the RAS－SOS1 interaction[J]. Proceedings of the National Academy of Sciences of the United States of America, 2019, 116（7）.

[113] XUE J Y, ZHAO Y, ARONOWITZ J, et al. Rapid non-uniform adaptation to conformation-specific KRAS（G12C）inhibition. [J]. Nature, 2020, 577（7790）.

[114] WELSCH M E, KAPLAN A, CHAMBERS J M, et al. Multivalent small-molecule Pan-RAS inhibitors[J]. Cell, 2017, 168（5）: 878-889.

[115] MAURER T, GARRENTON L S, ANGELA O H, et al. Small-molecule ligands bind to a distinct pocket in Ras and inhibit SOS-mediated nucleotide exchange activity[J]. Proceedings

of the National Academy of Sciences of the United States of America, 2012, 109（14）: 5299-5304.

[116] ZHANG J, ZHANG F, NIU R. Functions of Shp2 in cancer[J]. Journal of Cellular & Molecular Medicine, 2015, 19（9）.

[117] RASTOGI R, JIANG Z, AHMAD N, et al. Rapamycin induces mitogen-activated protein （MAP）kinase phosphatase-1（MKP-1）expression through activation of protein kinase B and mitogen-activated protein kinase kinase pathways[J]. Journal of Biological Chemistry, 2013, 288（47）: 33966-33977.

[118] SVEJDA B, KIDD M, KAZBEROUK A, et al. Limitations in small intestinal neuroendocrine tumor therapy by mTor kinase inhibition reflect growth factor‐mediated PI3K feedback loop activation via ERK1/2 and AKT[J]. Cancer, 2011, 117（18）: 4141-4154.

[119] YIZHOU Z, XIAOFANG T, QUAN W, et al. Attenuation of everolimus-induced cytotoxicity by a protective autophagic pathway involving ERK activation in renal cell carcinoma cells[J]. Drug Design Development & Therapy, 2018, 12: 911-920.

[120] AHMET Z; RYMA B, SHAH R H, et al. Erratum: Mutational landscape of metastatic cancer revealed from prospective clinical sequencing of 10 000 patients[J]. Nature Medicine, 2017, 23（8）: 703-713.

[121] NAGASAKA M, LI Y, SUKARI A, et al. KRAS G12C game of thrones, which direct KRAS inhibitor will claim the iron throne[J]. Cancer Treatment Reviews, 2020, 84: 101974.

[122] CHRISTENSEN J G, HALLIN J, ENGSTROM L D, et al. The KRAS inhibitor MRTX849 provides insight toward therapeutic susceptibility of KRAS-mutant cancers in mouse models and patients. [J]. Cancer Discovery, 2020, 10（1）: 54-71.

[123] CUTSEM E, HUIJBERTS S, GROTHEY A, et al. Binimetinib, encorafenib, and cetuximab triplet therapy for patients with BRAF V600E-mutant metastatic colorectal cancer: safety lead-in results from the Phase III BEACON colorectal cancer study[J]. Journal of clinical oncology: official journal of the American Society of Clinical Oncology, 2019, 37（17）.

[124] XUE J Y, ZHAO Y, ARONOWITZ J, et al. Rapid non-uniform adaptation to conformation-specific KRAS（G12C）inhibition. [J]. Nature, 2020, 577（7790）.

[125] SCHWARTZ P A, KUZMIC P, SOLOWIEJ J, et al. Covalent EGFR inhibitor analysis reveals importance of reversible interactions to potency and mechanisms of drug resistance[J].

Proceedings of the National Academy of Sciences of the United States of America，2014，111 （1）：173–178.

[126] YAEGER R，YAO Z，HYMAN D M，et al. Mechanisms of acquired resistance to BRAF V600E inhibition in colon cancers converge on RAF dimerization and are sensitive to its inhibition[J]. Cancer research，2017，77（23）：6513–6523.

[127] DOUGLAS B J，ALEXANDER M M，LISA Z，et al. Acquired BRAF inhibitor resistance： A multicenter meta–analysis of the spectrum and frequencies，clinical behaviour，and phenotypic associations of resistance mechanisms [J]. European Journal of Cancer，2015，51 （18）：2792–2799.

[128] BEAN J，BRENNAN C，SHIH J Y，et al. MET amplification occurs with or without T790M mutations in EGFR mutan t lung tumors with acquired resistance to gefitinib or erlotinib[J]. Proceedings of the National Academy of Sciences of the United States of America，2007，104 （52）：20932–20937.

[129] NAZARIAN R，SHI H，WANG Q，et al. Melanomas acquire resistance to B–RAF（V600E） inhibition by RTK or N–RAS upregulation[J]. Nature，2010，468（7326）：973–977.

[130] JESSIE V，JEFFREY R I，CLEMENS K，et al. Concurrent MEK2 mutation and BRAF amplification confer resistance to BRAF and MEK inhibitors in melanoma[J]. Cell Reports， 2013，4（6）：1090–1099.

[131] SHALEM O，SANJANA N E，ZHANG F. High–throughput functional genomics using CRISPR‒Cas9[J]. Nature Reviews Genetics，2015，16（5）：299–311.

[132] JIANG F，TAYLOR D W，CHEN J S，et al. Structures of a CRISPR–Cas9 R–loop complex primed for DNA cleavage[J]. Science，2016，351（6275）：867–871.

[133] DAHLMAN J E，ABUDAYYEH O O，JOUNG J，et al. Orthogonal gene knockout and activation with a catalytically active Cas9 nuclease[J]. Nature Biotechnology，2015，33（11）： 1159.

[134] TOH T B，LIM J J，CHOW K H. Epigenetics in cancer stem cells[J]. Molecular Cancer， 2017，16（1）：29.

[135] PANTSAR T. The current understanding of KRAS protein structure and dynamics[J]. Computational and Structural Biotechnology Journal，2020，18.

[136] NUSSINOV R，JANG H，TSAI C J. The structural basis for cancer treatment decisions[J]. Oncotarget，2014，5（17）：7285–302.

[137] HELEN, ADDERLEY, FIONA, et al. KRAS-mutant non-small cell lung cancer:
      Converging small molecules and immune checkpoint inhibition [J]. Ebiomedicine, 2019,
      41: 711-716.

[138] CUI W, FRANCHINI F, ALEXANDER M, et al. Real world outcomes in KRAS G12C
      mutation positive non-small cell lung cancer[J]. Lung Cancer, 2020, 146: 310-317.

[139] KARACHALIOU N, MAYO C, COSTA C, et al. KRAS mutations in lung cancer[J].
      Clinical Lung Cancer, 2013, 14 (3): 205-214.

[140] FENG H, ZHANG Y, BOS P H, et al. K-RasG12D has a potential allosteric small
      molecule binding site[J]. Biochemistry, 2019, 58 (21).

[141] LAMBA S, RUSSO M, SUN C, et al. RAF suppression synergizes with MEK inhibition in
      KRAS mutant cancer cells[J]. Cell Report, 2014, 8 (5): 1475-1483.

[142] BERTIN S, SAMSON M, PONS C, et al. Comparative proteomics study reveals that
      bacterial CpG motifs induce tumor cell autophagy in vitro and in vivo[J]. Molecular & Cellular
      Proteomics, 2008, 7 (12): 2311-2322.

[143] LINDSEY D S, ROBERTSON K M, PITTS T M, et al. Combined inhibition of MEK and
      aurora a kinase in KRAS/PIK3CA double-mutant colorectal cancer models[J]. Frontiers in
      Pharmacology, 2015, 6: 120.

[144] PEDRO, TORRES A, JOHN, et al. Shipping out MEK inhibitor resistance with SHP2
      inhibitors[J]. Cancer Discovery, 2018, 8 (10): 1210-1212.

[145] RODON J, DIENSTMANN R, SERRA V, et al. Development of PI3K inhibitors: lessons
      learned from early clinical trials[J]. Nature Reviews Clinical Oncology, 2013, 10 (3):
      143-153.

[146] DURRANT, DAVID E. Targeting the Raf kinases in human cancer: the Raf dimer
      dilemma[J]. British Journal of Cancer, 2018, 118 (7574): 3-8.

[147] STRICKLER J, FAKIH M, PRICE T, et al. SO-24 AMG 510, a novel small molecule
      inhibitor of KRAS G12C, for patients with advanced gastrointestinal cancers: Results
      from the CodeBreak 100 phase 1 trial[J]. Annals of Oncology, 2020, 31 (Supl. 3):
      S226-S226.

[148] PATRICELLI M P, JANES M R, LI L S, et al. Selective inhibition of oncogenic KRAS
      output with small molecules targeting the inactive state[J]. Cancer Discovery, 2016: 2159-
      8290.

[149] PIRO，LITO，MARTHA，et al.　Allele-specific inhibitors inactivate mutant KRAS G12C by a trapping mechanism．[J]．Science，2016，351（6273）：604-608．

[150] HANSEN，RASMUS，PETERS，et al.　The reactivity-driven biochemical mechanism of covalent KRASG12C inhibitors[J]．Nat Struct Mol Biol，2018，25（14）：454-462．

第二部分

CRISPR-Cas 系统的功能和应用

摘　要

CRISPR（clustered regularly interspaced short palindromic repeats）-Cas（CRISPR-asscociated）系统是在细菌和古细菌中发现的一种获得性免疫系统。从该系统的发现到作为一种基因编辑技术在生物体上进行研究应用经历了三十多年的时间。CRISPR-Cas系统能够精准的编辑靶向序列，实现特定基因的突变，目的序列的插入，以及定向单碱基突变，使得癌症的治疗成为可能，多种单基因或多基因遗传病的治疗得已实现，病毒引发的疾病得以一一攻克。这是本世纪医学研究和临床治疗上最重要的一项研究，也是人类攻克各种疾病的希望。本章内容主要描述了CRISPR-Cas系统的发现和探索历程，结构功能的研究，作用机制的发现，以及在肿瘤免疫疗法和其他医学领域的研究和应用。

【关键词】CRISPR-Cas；基因编辑；癌症治疗

Abstract

CRISPR （clustered regularly interspaced short palindromic repeats）–Cas （CRISPR–associated） system has been discovered as an aquired immunity system in bacterial and archaea. It took over–30–years' research from the discovery to its application as a gene editing technique in organics. CRISPR–Cas system can precisely edit the targeted sequences, such as achieving specific gene mutation and target gene insertion. This technology has been utilized in the treatment of cancer, single–gene or multi–genes genetic diseases, as well as viral diseases. It is one of the most important and popular discoveries in medical research and clinical development of this century, and it also holds promise for mankind to overcome various diseases. This chapter mainly describes the process of the discovery and exploration of the CRISPR–Cas system, the structure, function， and mechanism, as well as the recent advances and applications of CRISPR–Cas System in general cancer management, cancer immunotherapy, and other medical fields.

[Keywords] CRISPR–Cas; gene editing; cance therapy

CRISPR-Cas是clustered regularly interspaced short palindromic repeats – CRISPR-associated（Cas）的缩写，指的是成簇规律性间隔短回文重复序列及其相关序列。这一系统来源于细菌和古细菌的天然获得性免疫系统[1]。CRISPR是一段高度保守的间隔重复序列，Cas基因是编码Cas蛋白来行使剪切DNA功能的核酸内切酶[2]。这一系统的发现以及后续在真核生物尤其是哺乳动物上的成功利用使基因精准编辑成为可能[3]。基因编辑是指对基因组特定位置进行删除，插入或者定向改变基因序列的一种方法。CRIPSR-Cas系统进行基因编辑是目前最为简单且有效的，它是依赖于单链指导RNA（single guide RNA，sgRNA）引导特定的核酸内切酶在靶向DNA片段进行编辑。相比于利用人工介导的锌指核酸内切酶（zinc-finger nucleases，ZFNs）和类转录激活因子效应物核酸酶（transcription activator-like effector nucleases，TALENs）进行基因编辑，这项技术更精准、高效和节约成本。然而，CRISPR-Cas系统的发现、研究、应用与不断突破也经历了三十多年的漫长历程。本部分将详细介绍CRISPR-Cas系统的探索过程。

1　CRISPR-Cas系统的探索与发现

CRISPR-Cas系统是现在生命科学领域研究最为火热的基因编辑技术，因其简单，高效，适用范围广而被世界范围内的科研人员所青睐，广泛的应用于基础科研研究、临床治疗、植物及真菌的研究等。研究工作者也寄希望于应用此技术的靶向编辑来治疗各种癌症等人类疾病，改善农作物的产量、质量及抗性等性状。对于这一系统的研究，我们要追溯到三十多年前，始于对寄居于人类肠道细菌的研究（图1.1）。

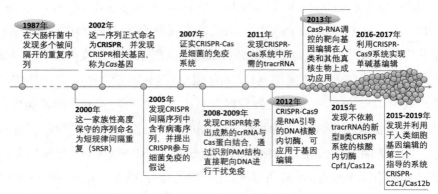

图 1.1　CRISPR-Cas 系统的研究进程

1987年，日本科学家石野良纯（Ishino Yoshizumi）等人在研究大肠杆菌（*Escherichia coli*）的*iap*基因时发现，*iap*基因3'端连有一段以前研究中从未发现的特殊的DNA序列。这段DNA序列包含多个29bp长的重复序列，这些重复序列并未首尾相连，而是被没有规律的DNA片段间隔开来，同时这段重复序列中有部分片段是反向互补的[4]（图1.2）。

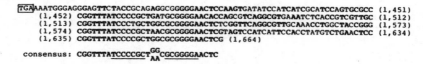

图 1.2　*iap* 基因 3' 端区域由 61 对碱基组成的重复序列的对比

底部序列显示了29个高度保守的核苷酸，其中包含14个反向互补的碱基（下划线所示）。方框内所示*iap*基因的终止密码子，括号内表示的是核酸位置。[4]

随着这一特殊序列的揭示，更多的研究发现在其他品系的大肠杆菌、其他的细菌、放线菌以及古细菌——地中海嗜盐菌（*Haloferax mediterranei*）中也发现了含有"重复-间隔-重复"特征的DNA片段[5-11]。经过十多年的研究，科学家在越来越多的原核生物中发现了这样特殊的DNA片段。到2000年，这样的间隔重复序列在40%左右的细菌和90%左右的古细菌中存在。西班牙阿利坎特大学（University of Alicante）的Farncisco Mojica等人在其发表的文章中将这一家族性高度保守的DNA序列命名为短规律间隔重复（short regularly spaced repeat，SRSR）[12]。

2002年，荷兰乌得勒支大学（Utrecht University）的Ruud Jansen实验室通过生物信息学分析发现这种特殊的DNA序列在不同物种中的重复序列碱基数存在差异，在21—37bp之间，如鼠伤寒沙门氏菌（*Salmonella typhimurium*）中的重复序列为21bp，化脓性链球菌（*Streptococcus pyogenes*）则为37，而这一特征序列只存在于细菌和古细菌中，不存在于真核生物和病毒中。同时Jansen与Mojica交流后，把这种串联重复序列正式命名为成簇间隔规律性短回文重复序列（Clustered regularly short palindromic repeats，CRISPR）[13]。詹森等人研究发现，在大多数真核生物中存在两个及以上的不同CRISPR序列，每一CRISPR位点附近始终存在着一段基因序列，这一序列与CRISPR基因存在着功能相关性，因此被称为CRISPR相关基因（CRISPR-associated genes，Cas）。在Jansen等人的研究中，他们发现了4个*cas*基因，并命名为*cas1*，*cas2*，*cas3*，*cas4*。他们指出Cas1和Cas2蛋白的功能还未确定，但Cas3具有解旋酶活性，Cas4蛋白的功能与核酸外切酶相似。此后，这个在原核生物中存在的特殊的DNA重复序列CRISPR以及其相邻的*cas*基因正式进入了科学家们的视线，而且也预测其功能是参与DNA的修复和基因表达调控过程[14-15]。

2005年是推动CRISPR研究进展的重要一年，Alexander Bolotin，Gilles Vergnaud和Francisco Mojica三位科学家领导的实验室，在同一年分别发表文章，指出CRISPR中的间隔序列（Spacer）与侵染细菌的病毒或噬菌体具有很高的同源性，说明细菌体内含有的许多间隔序列来源于病毒或者噬菌体[1, 16-17]。其中Mojica实验室发现病毒无法感染携带有与病毒同源的间隔序列的细菌，而可以入侵那些不含有与病毒同源的间隔序列的细菌，由此他们推测CRISPR系统可能与细菌的免疫防御机制有关[16]。结合对CRISPR的转录组研究发现[18]和对*cas*基因编码的蛋白可能是核酸酶和解旋酶结构域的推断[2, 13, 17, 19]，有研究人员提出，CRISPR-Cas系统是使用反义RNA作为过去的入侵记忆来实现自身的免疫防御[20]。

CRISPR-Cas系统在细菌体内起到免疫防御的功能在2007年得到了证实。

Rodolphe Barrango用嗜热链球菌（*Streptococcus thermophilus*）和噬菌体开展了一系列的实验。他将链球菌和噬菌体放在一起，大部分的链球菌会被噬菌体杀掉，只有一小部分存活下来。Barrango对这些存活下来的链球菌进行了分析，发现链球菌的间隔序列中含有噬菌体基因组片段，因此，可以对病毒的再次入侵产生抗性。人为的去除这一特定序列后会影响链球菌的抗性表现。因此，他们认为链球菌能够通过 CRISPR-Cas系统，将噬菌体的DNA片段整合到自身基因组中成为新的间隔片段，从而抵抗噬菌体的再次入侵，而且其抗性的特异性取决于CRISPR中的间隔序列。同时，有研究发现，细菌的这种获得性免疫是可以遗传的[1]。这一研究发现支持了我们的理论基础，乳制品行业中使用的培养细菌存在天然CRISPR-Cas系统可以对噬菌体产生免疫，这是CRISPR-Cas系统在生物技术上的首次成功应用[21]。细菌利用CRISPR-Cas系统来抵御病毒入侵的具体机制尚未清楚，但以后的研究逐渐解开了这个神秘而强大的系统的面纱。

2008年，荷兰瓦赫宁恩大学（Wageningen University & Research）的John等人通过研究大肠杆菌的CRISPR-Cas系统发现CRISPR序列可转录出成熟的RNA—CRISPR RNA（crRNA），crRNA与Cas蛋白结合干扰病毒在大肠杆菌的繁殖[22]。同一年，美国西北大学（Northwestern University）的Erik Sontheimer等则在对表皮葡萄球菌（*Staphylococcus epidermidis*）的CRISPR-Cas系统的研究中发现，其干扰机制是直接靶向DNA来限制致病菌中抗生素抗性的传播[23]。而病毒群体的广泛重组也可以避免与细菌CRISPR间隔序列的同源性，因此，只有短期获取的间隔序列才能有效地发挥识别作用[24]。2009年，Mojica实验室通过研究发现crRNA能够准确地定位到外来的DNA分子片段与自身某一间隔序列同源是依赖于一个在CRISPR-Cas系统中相对保守的结构PAMs（Photo-spacer adjacent motifs）[25]。PAMs通常只含有几个核苷酸，而且在不同的CRISPR-Cas系统是不同的[25-26]。

2011年，瑞典于默奥大学（Umeå University）的Emmanuelle Charpentier研究小组在分析人类病原体化脓性链球菌（*Streptococcus pyogenes*）的RNA序列的差异性时发现了一种与crRNA前体转录因子重复序列有24个核苷酸互补配对的反式编码小RNA，并称为tracrRNA（trans-activating crRNA）。tracrRNA通过与广泛保守的内源性RNA酶Ⅲ（RNaseⅢ）和CRISPR相关的Csn1蛋白的相互作用来指导crRNA的成熟。所有这些成分对保护化脓性链球菌免受噬菌体的侵染至关重要。他们的研究也第一个显示宿主因子（RNsaeⅢ）是细菌RNA介导免疫所必需的实例[27]。

随着对CRISPR-Cas系统在不同细菌和古细菌中的深入研究，一些同源的CRISPR相关蛋白在不同物种间参与免疫反应而命名不同，而且发现了更多的相关基因及表达蛋白参与反应，使CRISPR-Cas系统分类命名过于复杂。因此，美国国家卫生研究院（National Institutes of Health）的Eugene V. Koonin等人首次创建了一套统一而又灵活的分类方案，他们将CRISPR-Cas系统详细的划分成三个不同类型——Ⅰ类、Ⅱ类和Ⅲ类，包含10个亚类[28]。随着研究发现的Cas蛋白的增多，而后又多次对CRISPR-Cas系统的分类进行更新，我们会在后面章节详细讲解。

以上都是针对CRISPR-Cas系统在细菌或古细菌体内发挥免疫作用抵御病毒和质粒的入侵等领域的研究。CRISPR-Cas作为基因编辑工具被应用是在2012年被美国加州大学伯克利分校（University of California，Berkley）的Jennifer Doudna和瑞典于默奥大学的Emmanuelle Charpentier共同研究证实的。她们利用体外实验证明成熟的crRNA通过碱基互补配对与tracrRNA形成特殊的双链RNA结构，指导Cas9蛋白在目标片段切断双链DNA。在与crRNA互补的目标位点，Cas9蛋白的HNH核酸酶结构域和RuvC-like结构域会分别切割crRNA互补链和crRNA非互补链。当tracrRNA：crRNA的双链结构被设计成单条RNA嵌合体（single guide RNA，sgRNA）时，也可以指导Cas9蛋白切割目标DNA（图1.3）。她们的研究为我们揭示了利用双RNA结构引导的在特定位点切割的核酸内切酶家族，并提出了利用CRISPR-Cas系统进行基因编辑的巨大潜力[29]。Jennifer的研究还指出，CRISPR-Cas系统依靠RNA引导的特定位点识别和基因沉默与RNA干扰的作用效果相似，但作用机制却有别于RNA干扰[30]。Jennifer Doudna和Emmanuelle Charpentier这两位杰出的研究人员也因在CRISPR-Cas系统上的重大突破，获得了2020年的诺贝尔化学奖。

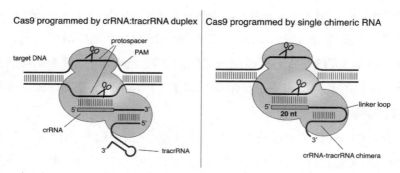

图 1.3   CRISPR-Cas9 系统可通过基因工程改造的 sgRNA 引导实现基因编辑

如图1.3所示，左图是在Ⅱ类CRISPR-Cas系统，Cas9受到两个RNA结构的引导，该结构是由促进crRNA成熟的tracrRNA和具有靶向功能的crRNA碱基互补配对构成。右图是将crRNA的3'端融合到tracrRNA的5'端产生的嵌合RNA引导Css9。[30]

将CRISPR-Cas系统作为基因编辑工具，应用到哺乳动物细胞中或植物及其他真核生物体内的大量研究报告从2013年开始接踵而至。麻省理工学院（Massachusetts Institute of Technology）张锋在2013年初，第一个发表文章证明这一系统能够成功应用到真核生物中进行基因编辑。他们证实cas9可以在小RNA的指导下，在人类及小鼠细胞的内源基因座进行精确剪切，同时他们将cas9改造成缺口酶促进同源修复。他们还将多个引导序列构建到单个CRISPR阵列中，实现了同时编辑多个基因位点[31]。他们的研究结果证实了利用RNA引导的核酸酶技术具有易操作性和广泛应用性。同年，哈佛大学（Harvard University）的George Church和加州大学旧金山分校（University of California，San Francisco）的Lei S.Qi（目前就职于斯坦福大学）也成功地将CRISPR-Cas系统成功应用到哺乳动物中[32-33]。Church实验室在秀丽隐杆线虫（*Caenorhabditis elegans*）上实现了用sgRNA引导Cas9准确定位目标序列，他们的实验为构建功能丧失型突变体提供了方便而有效的方法。Qi的研究团队则将Cas9蛋白改造成失去核酸内切酶活性的dCas9，通过引导RNA（gRNA）将dCas9融合到有独特功能的效应域上，可以有效地抑制或激活DNA的转录，dCas9与转录阻遏物的耦合可以沉默特定内源基因的表达，他们将其称为CRISPR干扰

（CRISPRinterference，CRISPRi）。他们构建的CRISPR系统能够引导蛋白结合到特定的DNA序列，揭示了CRISPRi作为常规工具在真核生物细胞中精确调控基因表达的潜力。

　　广泛应用于基因编辑的CRISPR-Cas9属于Ⅱ类CRISPR系统，只需要RNA介导核酸酶对特定序列进行剪切。通过基因工程构建的sgRNA是根据crRNA和tracrRNA互补配对后设计的，与Cas9核酸酶结合，指导其在识别位点剪辑靶向序列，但靶向序列附近必须有含NGG或NAG的PAM序列（图1.4）。

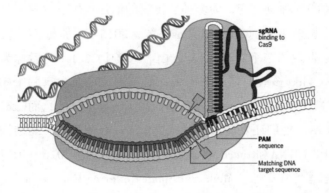

图 1.4　sgRNA 引导 Cas9 蛋白识别 PAM 序列在靶向位点进行基因编辑
此图片引用自参考文献[50]。

　　2015年，张锋实验室在*Cell*杂志发表文章，报道了一种不同于Cas9的新型Ⅱ类CRISPR效应因子Cpf1，也称作Cas12a。这是一个不依赖于tracrRNA而只由单个RNA介导的核酸内切酶，它通过识别富含胸腺嘧啶（T）的PAM序列靶向特定位点。Cas9在靶向位点剪切形成的是平末端，而Cpf1在靶向位点剪切后形成的是黏性末端。他们同时也证实CRISPR-Cpf1系统能够在人类细胞内进行基因编辑。识别这种干扰机制扩大了我们对CRISPR-Cas系统的理解，也促进了其基因编辑的应用[34]。

　　随着测序技术的不断发展以及在人类疾病研究上的应用，科学家们发现很多遗传性疾病都是由点突变引起的，即单个碱基发生改变从而引发疾病。之前的基因编辑技术都是在靶向位点剪切双链DNA而随机的引发片段缺失或插入，不能有效地进行单个碱基的编辑。2016年，哈佛大学的David R. Liu提出了一套不需要剪切双链DNA，能够靶向进行C→T或G→A的单碱基替换方法。他们设计了CRISPR-Cas9与胞苷脱氨酶的融合蛋白，这个融合蛋白保留了RNA指导的编辑能力，但不会诱导DNA断裂，同时介导胞苷直接转化成尿苷。这是一个可以在大约5个核苷酸窗口内进行胞苷转换的碱基编辑器[35]。一年后，他们这个研究团队又将腺嘌呤脱氨酶与CRISPR-Cas9系统融合，可以介导A和T到G或C的转换，在人体内的编辑效率超过了50%[36]。这个技术可以有效地纠正与人类疾病相关的各种点突变，为多种遗传病的治疗提供了有效工具。

为了探索更多未知的CRISPR-Cas系统，2015年，张锋实验室设计利用生物信息学方法发现了三个新型的Cas蛋白[37]。其中C2c1（之后称为Cas12b）和C2c3含有RuvC-like核酸内切酶结构域，而预测C2c2是含有两个HEPN RNA酶结构域的蛋白。C2c1调控crRNA成熟是依赖于traceRNA的，而C2c2的调控则不依赖于tracrRNA。他们还发现C2c1系统类似于Cpf1依赖于PAM结构干扰DNA，但同时依赖于crNRNA和tracrRNA进行靶向位点切割。2016—2017年，美国斯隆·凯特琳纪念癌症中心（Memorial Sloan Kettering Cancer Center）的杨辉实验室和中国科学院生物物理研究所的王艳丽课题组分别在Cell上发表文章，揭示了含有sgRNA的C2c1晶体结构与Cpf1和Cas9显著不同，在靶向序列的单个碱基突变后，C2c1核酸内切酶的剪切活性降低，这表明C2c1对靶向位点的序列要求极其严格[38-39]。2019年，张锋实验室发表文章称他们建立了继CRISPR-Cas9和CRISPR-Cas12a/Cpf1之后，第三个RNA指导的核酸酶剪切平台CRISPR-Cas12b/C2c1，用于人类细胞中的基因编辑[40]。

CRISPR-Cas9系统因为没有物种的限制，除了在哺乳动物上的成功应用外，也在植物和真菌上得到了广泛应用。研究人员利用CRISPR-Cas系统对人类遗传性疾病的治疗展开各项研究，并于2016年完成了第一个由CRISPR-Cas9编辑进行的临床治疗。CRISPR-Cas9系统在临床上的应用我们会在后面章节进行详细介绍。

2 CRISPR-Cas系统的结构组成及作用机理

2.1 CRISPR-Cas 系统的结构组成

随着深入的研究，科学家们已经了解了CRISPR-Cas系统的构成。CRISPR-Cas系统主要有两部分组成——CRISPR基因阵列和cas基因家族，分别执行不同的生理功能，CRISPR基因阵列包含了重复序列和间隔序列，以及一段前导序列，负责靶向序列的识别，cas基因有获得外源基因片段和剪切靶向序列的功能。该系统还包含一段tracrRNA序列（图2.1）。

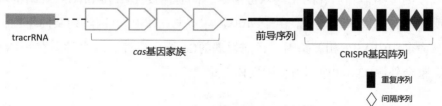

图 2.1　CRISPR-Cas 系统的基本构成

2.1.1　前导序列

前导序列位于CRISPR基因阵列的5'端，是一段富含A-T的、与转录有关的保守序列。这个序列包含启动子，用来启动CRISPR序列的转录。

2.1.2　CRISPR 基因阵列

CRISPR基因阵列由重复序列和间隔序列组成，这两种序列呈间隔排列，这也是CRISPR一词的创建缘由。重复序列在同一物种的细菌或古细菌中的碱基长度和组成是相对保守的，而在不同物种之间会存在较大差异[13]。间隔序列是由病毒或质粒的DNA片段衍生而来，用于识别特定的外源序列。由于间隔序列是来自于不同的外源生物，其序列长度和碱基组成差异较大[1, 21]。一般来说，重复序列的长度在21—37bp之间，间隔序列的长度则在30—40bp之间[13, 21]。重复序列对于间隔序列在CRISPR基因阵列中的位置和方向起决定性作用[41]。

2.1.3 *cas* 基因家族

*cas*基因家族是CRISPR基因阵列附近的一个基因簇，编码的蛋白具有核酸酶、解旋酶、聚合酶等活性，以及含有RNA结合蛋白特性的结构域[42]。Cas9蛋白是Cas家族中研究最多的一个蛋白，因为其参与的基因编辑系统只需要sgRNA和Cas9蛋白即可完成靶向位点的剪切。Cas9是一个含有两个核酸酶结构域的多功能蛋白，HNH和RuvC-like结构域[20]。Cas9利用HNH结构域切割与crRNA的20个核苷酸序列互补的DNA链；RuvC-like结构域切割与互补链碱基互补配对的DNA链（图2.1）[29, 43]。Cas9对于防御病毒入侵至关重要，负责切断入侵的噬菌体和质粒的靶向双链DNA，同时需要HNH和RuvC-like结构域干扰质粒的转化效率[27, 44-46]。由于*cas*基因家族与CRISPR基因阵列共同作用，因此被命名为CRISPR相关基因。目前发现的Cas蛋白已经有40多种，在crRNA成熟、整合外源DNA和序列剪切中发挥着重要作用[19]。

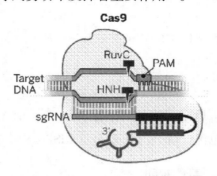

图 2.2　Cas9 蛋白的 HNH 结构域和 RuvC-like 结构域在进行
基因编辑时剪切靶向序列的双链 DNA[19]

此图片引用自参考文献[50]。

2.1.4　tracrRNA

反式激活crRNA—tracrRNA，是一种在化脓性链球菌中Ⅱ类CRISPR–Cas基因座上游被反编码的小RNA。它参与有核糖核酸酶Ⅲ和Cas9蛋白作用的crRNA成熟过程，并于成熟的crRNA形成双链结构指导核酸内切酶进行DNA双链切割，研究发现这一过程能够赋予细菌对外来入侵的特异性免疫反应（图1.3左图）[27, 29]。

2.2　CRISPR-Cas 系统的作用机理

CRISPR–Cas系统作为细菌的一种获得性免疫防御系统，其作用机制被科学家们深入的研究和探索。研究表明，CRISPR–Cas系统作用机理可大致分为三个阶段：获得，表达，干扰（图2.2）[1-2, 16-17, 20, 22-23, 41, 47-50]。

CRISPR–Cas系统的获得性免疫防御过程的第一阶段就是CRISPR的获得，即获得入侵者的一小段DNA，整合到CRISPR重复序列间的间隔序列（图2.2）。当病毒，质粒或者噬菌体等外源DNA入侵细菌时，Cas1和Cas2蛋白复合体识别并携带入侵者的一小段含有PAM序列的DNA向CRISPR基因阵列中添加一个间隔序列[44, 47]。间隔序列一端的PAM序列能够确保其以正确的方向插入到CRISPR基因列阵中[51-54]。PAM序列在间隔序列的获取和CRISPR系统的体外应用上都起着关键作用，不同的CRISPR–Cas系统的PAM识别序列也是不同的[25-26]。新的间隔序列被整合到前导序列与相邻的重复序列之间，使得CRISPR基因阵列中存有该入侵者的序列信息，这就形成了细菌感染的遗传记忆。

表达阶段是CRISPR基因阵列表达产生成熟crRNA的过程。当病毒、质粒或者噬菌体等外源DNA再次感染细菌时，在前导序列的调控下，CRISPR被转录为含有重复序列和间隔序列的长crRNA前体（pre-crRNA），*cas*基因家族转录翻译成Cas蛋白将形成具有切割功能的复合物。由于crRNA前体含有回文重复序列，因此会形成一系列的发夹结构。随后crRNA前体在Cas蛋白等核酸内切酶的作用下被加工成短的含单一间隔序列的成熟crRNA。不同类型的CRISPR-Cas系统中参与crRNA成熟过程的Cas蛋白也不同，即使不同类型的CRISPR-Cas系统同时存在，它们也不会相互参与crRNA前体的加工过程[55]。

　　CRISPR-Cas系统对靶向序列的干扰原理是与Cas蛋白结合的crRNA定位与之碱基互补配的序列以触发靶向位点的降解，序列降解的过程是通过特定的Cas核酸酶进行的（图2.2）[22, 28]。不同CRISPR-Cas类型的特点和Cas蛋白在获得性免疫过程中的作用将会在下一章节详细介绍。

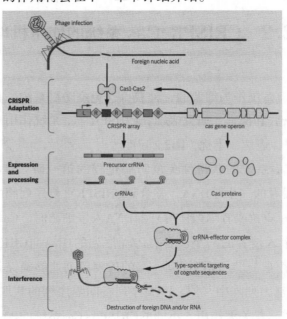

图 2.2　CRISPR-Cas 系统的获得性免疫防御过程 [22, 28]

3 CRISPR-Cas系统的分类

　　CRISPR-Cas系统的命名经过了两次变更。2011年，美国国家卫生研究院（National Institutes of Health）的Eugene V. Koonin等人首次创建了一套统一的分类方案，他们将CRISPR-Cas系统详细的划分成三个不同类型（Type）——Ⅰ类、Ⅱ类和Ⅲ类，包含10个亚类（Subtype）[28]。CRISPR-Cas系统进化迅速，尤其表现在多位点重排和单模块的水平移动。这些变化直接使系统发育分类变得复杂化。Eugene等人于2015年发表文章称他们采用两步分类方法，首先确定每个CRISPR-Cas基因位点中的所有cas基因，然后确定特征基因和独特基因的结构，根据这些基因位点划分类型和亚类，因此，将大多数的CRISPR-Cas基因位点划分为不同的种类（Class）、类型（Type）和亚类（Subtype）[42]。新的分类保留了先前版本的整体结构，并扩展到含有2个大的种类，6个小的类型，16个亚类。2017年，Eugene与张锋、Kira S. Makarova在Cell杂志上发表了CRISPR-Cas系统的两大种类的快照，详细介绍了种类组成，相应Cas蛋白结构，以及作用机制等[56]。而后Eugene等研究学者又于2018年和2020年根据新的研究发现对该系统的分类进行了补充与完善[57, 65-66]。

　　CRISPR-Cas的种类1系统是利用具有包含多个Cas蛋白的多蛋白效应复合物和引导RNA共同作用获得性免疫反应，而种类2系统的特点是其效应因子是单个的多结构域蛋白（图3.1）。cas1和cas2是CRISPR-Cas系统普遍存在的两个基因，它们转录翻译形成的蛋白复合体在外源基因获得阶段能够将新的间隔序列插入到CRISPR基因阵列中。cas4基因则在两个种类中的部分类型中存在，而tracrRNA序列只存于种类2的部分类型中。

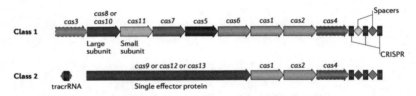

图 3.1　CRISPR-Cas 系统的两个不同种类的基本组成

3.1　CRISPR-Cas 系统——种类 1

种类1包含了三个类，分别是 Ⅰ 类、Ⅲ类和Ⅳ类[57]（图3.2）。

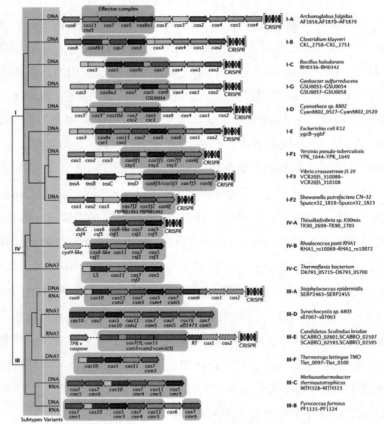

图 3.2　CRISPR-Cas 系统种类 1 的具体分类

如图3.2所示，图中同源基因用相同颜色标注，未知功能的基因用灰色表示。橘色阴影显示的是该系统的效应因子模块。Ⅲ–B、Ⅲ–C、Ⅲ–E、Ⅲ–F、Ⅳ–B和Ⅳ–C亚类基因座缺少了CRISPR基因阵列。图3.2右边的一列表示含有该系统的细菌或古细菌，以及相应的基因范围。（引自Kira S. Makarova et al，2020）

　　Ⅰ类系统包含了特征基因cas3以及其变体cas3'，它编码单链DNA刺激的家族2解旋酶，能解旋双链DNA和DNA–RNA双链结构。通常解旋酶结构域与参与靶向DNA切割的HD家族核酸内切酶结构域融合。一般情况下，HD结构域位于Cas3蛋白的氨基酸末端或由单独的与cas3'临近的cas3"基因编码。Ⅰ类系统又被分成7个亚类，分为Ⅰ–A到Ⅰ–G，Ⅰ–F则分成Ⅰ–F1、Ⅰ–F2和Ⅰ–F3。Ⅰ–C到Ⅰ–F亚类的CRISPR–Cas系统通常由单个操纵子编码，该操纵子包含cas1，cas2和cas3基因以及编码Cas复合体亚基的基因。Ⅰ–A和Ⅰ–B亚类基因座含有不同的组合，其中cas基因聚集在两个或多个操纵子中[28, 58-59]。cas4基因在Ⅰ类系统里不存在于Ⅰ–E亚类和Ⅰ–F亚类，cas3基因在Ⅰ–F亚类中是与cas2基因融合在一起的。cas8基因在Ⅰ类的大多数亚类中都存在，但却存在很大的差异性，即使在同一亚类中，cas8基因也表现出不同家族。尽管基因的进化过程较复杂，但我们可以认识到Ⅰ–B亚类与Ⅰ类的祖先组成最为接近。cas8b1基因的出现定义了Ⅰ–B亚类的一个子类，在古细菌CRISPR–Cas系统分类中被定义为Ⅰ–G亚类[59]。

　　Ⅲ类系统的特征基因是cas10，它编码含有多个结构域的蛋白。Cas10蛋白包含一个Palm结构域，与许多核酸聚合酶和环化酶核心结构域同源，是Ⅲ类crRNA效应复合物的最大亚基。Ⅲ类CRISRP–Cas系统又被分为六个不同的亚类，Ⅲ–A到Ⅲ–F。Cas10蛋白在不同的Ⅲ类系统中普遍存在，但也显示出广泛的序列差异，Cas5和Cas7蛋白也是所有Ⅲ类系统中都含有的小亚基蛋白。通常HD家族核酸酶结构域也会与Cas10蛋白融合，但该结构域有别于跟Ⅰ类Cas蛋白结合的结构域，它含有一个保守的环形排列的基序[14, 20]。Ⅲ–A和Ⅲ–B亚类是通过含有不同的小亚基csm2和cmr5来区分的，Ⅲ–A亚类基因座通常包含cas6基因，而大多数Ⅲ–B基因座缺乏该基因[28, 59]。另外两个亚类Ⅲ–C和Ⅲ–D分别由Ⅲ-B和Ⅲ-A演变而来，这两个亚类都不含有*cas1*和*cas2*基因，可能会引起反式的间隔序列整合。Ⅲ-C的显著特征是Cas10环化酶样的结构域序列变异，失去活性。Ⅲ-D亚类的Cas10蛋白缺少HD结构域。Ⅲ-E则是由多种Cas7蛋白和一个假定的Csm2-like小亚基融合组成，与crRNA结合的效应因子被压缩在单个体积较大的多结构域蛋白中，这使Ⅲ-E亚类与种类2系统相似。但通过对结构域和序列的分析可以明确的将这一亚类归到种类1中。Ⅲ-F亚类含有的Cas5和Cas7，以及效应因子复合体与其他Ⅲ类系统具有相似性，而其所含的一个小亚基表现出该亚类的独特性[66]。Ⅲ类CRISPR-Cas系统特征基因的*cas10*的发展演化过程与该类亚基的分类是一致的，每个亚基都代表了一个独特的进化分支[42, 58-59]。

CRISPR-Cas系统的Ⅳ则分成3个亚类，分别是Ⅳ-A、Ⅳ-B和Ⅳ-C。这三个亚基都含有Cas5和Cas7蛋白，但不含有Cas1和Cas2蛋白，而且Cas基因家族不与CRSIPR基因阵列相邻，因此，在很多情况下是在没有CRISPR基因表达的基因组中编码蛋白的。Ⅳ-B亚类是Ⅳ-A的变体，它不含有*dinG*基因，但预测含有效应因子复合物的小亚基的不同形式，大多数Ⅳ-B亚类的基因座中含有辅助基因*cysH*。Ⅳ-C亚类与其他两个Ⅳ类亚类不同的是推测该亚类的大亚基含有HD核酸酶结构域，可以切割目标DNA[59, 66]。

3.2　CRISPR-Cas 系统——种类 2

这一种类同样包含了3个不同类型，Ⅱ类、Ⅴ类和Ⅵ类，以及17个亚类[57, 66]（图3.3）。Ⅰ，Ⅱ，Ⅲ类系统是最早被系统划分的三个类型，而Ⅱ类系统完全有别于Ⅰ类和Ⅲ类，是最简单的CRISPR-Cas系统，因此，成为目前研究和应用最为广泛的基因编辑工具。

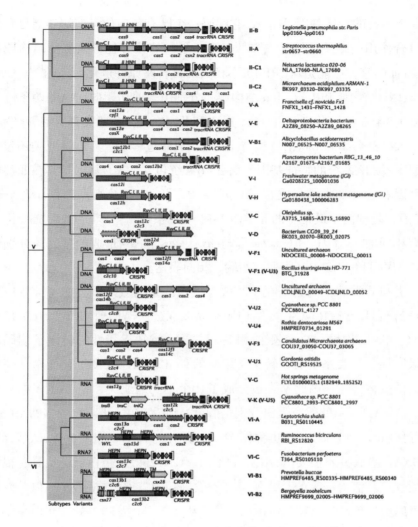

图 3.3　CRISPR-Cas 系统种类 2 的具体分类

如图3.3所示，图中同源基因用相同颜色标注。*cas1*和*cas2*基因作为单个亚基存在于 V-D、VI-A 和 VI-D 亚类，在分类图中用虚线表示。效应蛋白的结构域用不同颜色表示：RuvC-like核酸酶用绿色，HNH核酸酶用黄色，HEPN（higher eukaryotes and prokaryotes nucleotide-binding）RNA酶用紫色，跨膜结构域用蓝色。图3.3右边的一列表示含有该系统的细菌或古细菌，以及相应的基因范围。

Ⅱ类系统的特征基因是*cas9*，它编码一个既有靶向位点剪切功能也有外源基因整合作用的多结构域蛋白[60-61]。Cas9蛋白的核心包含核酸酶结构域和富含Arg特征的簇，可能是从CRISPR不相关的可转座原件进化而来的[62]。Cas9蛋白含有HNH结构域和RuvC-like结构域，分别用来剪切靶向DNA的两条链。Ⅱ类又分为3个亚类，分别是Ⅱ-A、Ⅱ-B和Ⅱ-C。这3个亚类都含有*cas1*和*cas2*基因，大多都会编码tracrRNA参与crRNA的成熟过程[62-64]。Ⅱ-A亚类还包含了*csn2*基因，是该系统的特征基因，而Ⅱ-B系统包含的*cas4*基因是其在Ⅱ类中的特征基因。Ⅱ-C亚类被分成Ⅱ-C1和Ⅱ-C2，Ⅱ-C1系统则只含有*cas1*，*cas2*和*cas9*基因，是细菌中最常见的Ⅱ类CRISPR-Cas系统[62-63]。Ⅱ-C2系统跟Ⅱ-B系统含有相同的*cas*基因，但*cas9*基因与*cas1*，*cas2*和*cas4*形成的基因簇分别位于tracrRNA序列和CRISPR基因列阵两端，相向表达。

Ⅴ类与Ⅱ类的不同之处在于其效应蛋白的结构域。Ⅴ类的特征效应蛋白是Cas12，它只含有RuvC-like结构域来完成双链DNA的剪切[67-68]。Cas12蛋白的RuvC-like结构域与TnpB蛋白相关，它是一类缺乏特性的转座子编码的蛋白超级家族。Ⅴ类系统通过转座子编码的TnpB核酸酶反复进化而来，并产生了大量的变体[73-75]，因此Ⅴ类被分成了10个不同的亚类，Ⅴ-A到Ⅴ-I，以及Ⅴ-U。Ⅴ-A到Ⅴ-I的效应蛋白分别是Cas12a到Cas12f。研究比较多的是Cas12a（也称作Cpf1）和Cas12b（也称作C2c1）蛋白。Cas12a蛋白与crRNA结合靶向特定DNA位点，并不需要tracrRNA的参与。Cas12b效应蛋白被证实具有很强的干扰活性[76]。值得一提的是，Ⅴ-F亚类含有Cas12f（之前称为Cas14）效应蛋白，可以剪切单链DNA和双链DNA[70-71]，Ⅴ-G亚类的Cas12g效应蛋白是RNA引导的RNA酶，也同时具有RNA酶和DNA酶活性[72]。

Ⅵ类是第一个也是迄今为止唯一只切割单链RNA的CRISPR-Cas系统。Ⅵ类的特征效应蛋白是Cas13，它与Cas9和Cas12不同，它含有两个间隔很远的HEPN（higher eukaryotes and prokaryotes nucleotide-binding）结构域，这个结构域广泛的存在于不同的免疫系统，用来靶向外来DNA的转录序列。Cas13蛋白还显示出靶向识别触发的非特异性RNA酶活性，并诱导有病毒感染的细菌休眠[69]。Ⅵ类被分成了4个亚类，Ⅳ-A到Ⅳ-D，对应的效应蛋白是Cas13a到

Cas13d。这一类型，尤其是Ⅵ-A亚类系统已经被研究利用到人类和植物体内RNA靶向失活的研究，相对于RNA干扰技术，CRISPR-Cas13a被证实具有与RNAi相似的效率，但具有更高的特异性[77]。

4 CRISPR-Cas9基因编辑技术在抗肿瘤免疫治疗中的应用

　　基因编辑技术的不断创新推进了医学在基因层面的研究。在CRISPR-Cas9技术出现之前，只能通过同源基因重组，对庞大的变异体库进行筛选以及体细胞核移植技术来完成DNA的编辑以及特定基因的改造。在自然情况下同源基因重组技术效率极低，变异体库的筛选以及体细胞核移植技术耗时耗力，极大地限制了研究的进展以及医学临床应用。这几种方法的限制性使研究人员不断寻找更高效简便的基因编辑方法。

4.1　基因编辑技术的研究进展

　　基因编辑是一种能够比较精准地对生物体特定基因位点进行修饰的一项技术。起初，研究人员利用人工核酸内切酶（engineered endonuclease，EEN）介导的基因定点编辑技术，该技术能够在修饰位点诱导产生DNA双链断裂（double strain break，DSB）和重连实现基因序列改变。通过人工核酸内切酶介导的 DSB，基因突变的概率大于1%，有时甚至超过50%，因此，人工核酸内切酶被称为"DNA剪刀"。人工核酸内切酶经过不断改良由一代的"DNA剪刀"——锌指核酸内切酶（zinc finger endonuclease，ZFN）也逐渐发展为第二代"DNA剪刀"——类转录激活因子效应物核酸酶（transcription activator –like effector nuclease，TALEN），这两代"DNA剪刀"都是由DNA结合蛋白与核酸内切酶 FokⅠ融合而成。虽然人工核酸内切酶技术使基因编辑技术更高效简便，但人工核酸内切酶制备复杂，成本昂贵，在基因编辑技术应用上无法进行大规模的基因筛选，所以也拥有一定的局限性。CRISPR-Cas9系统的发现，使基因编辑技术有了突飞猛进的发展。研究人员将tracrRNA-crRNA双链RNA改造成sgRNA，与Cas9蛋白组合即可完成靶向序列的剪切，sgRNA-Cas9复合体进入细胞核并识别PAM序列，在其后方3个碱基的地方切断DNA，并产生平末端切口。借助非同源末端连接（non homologous end-joining，NHEJ）机制或同源修复（homologous direct repair，HDR）机制进行修复[49]（图4.1）。非同源末端连接可诱导断裂的双链DNA重连，引起基因片段的插入或缺失，使基因的功能改变或丧失。同源修复则是利用模板DNA进行同源重组修复，实现目标序列的插入。CRISPR-Cas9技术较前两代利用人工核酸内切酶进行基因编辑的原理更加简单，更具有独特性和灵活性。CRISPR-Cas9系统是目前基因编辑领域研究和应用最为广泛的技术，它被应用于生物学及医学的各种领域中，如基因表达，动物模型的构建，基因治疗，肿瘤抑制等。尤其在肿瘤免疫治疗中，取得了很大的研究进展。

免疫治疗是一种靶向性强、副作用小的恶性肿瘤治疗方法。肿瘤免疫治疗是一种应用免疫学的原理和方法对肿瘤疾病进行特异性治疗的方法，该方法通过主动或被动方式提高肿瘤细胞的免疫原性和对效应细胞杀伤的敏感性，激活抗肿瘤免疫应答，并通过免疫细胞和效应分子进入到宿主体内，协同机体免疫系统对肿瘤细胞的生长起到杀伤或抑制作用。当异物入侵机体时会激发机体的免疫系统，机体会分泌抗体来阻挡异物入侵，而肿瘤细胞会诱导机体抑制机体免疫系统的正常功能，肿瘤免疫治疗就是通过阻断肿瘤的这种抑制作用，恢复机体的正常免疫系统，最终控制和杀伤肿瘤细胞。根据免疫机制的不同，肿瘤免疫治疗主要分为两类。第一类是抗体靶向疗法，通过采用相应的靶向药物对肿瘤生长所需的特定分子的靶点结合来抑制肿瘤细胞的生长。第二类是过继免疫疗法，首先获取患者体内的免疫细胞，在体外诱导出对肿瘤有杀伤或抑制作用的细胞，再输入到患者体内进行抗肿瘤作用。

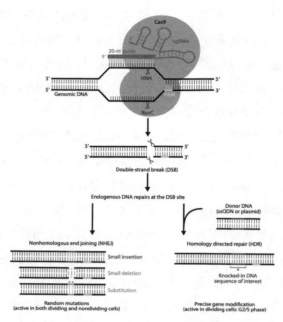

图 4.1 CRISPR-Cas9 介导的基因编辑机制

此图片引用自参考文献[49]。

4.2 在免疫检查点抑制剂（immune checkpoint inhibitor）阻断疗法上的应用

利用单克隆抗体共靶向的免疫检查点抑制性已在多种恶性肿瘤中表现出临床活性[78]。免疫检查点，例如PD-1（程序性死亡分子）和CTLA-4（和细胞毒T淋巴细胞相关抗原4），作为抑制T细胞反应的抑制分子以及免疫反应的负调节因子会直接影响T细胞的活性，导致机体的免疫机制对肿瘤细胞失去作用。在免疫检查点抑制剂中，PD-1和CTLA-4抑制剂表现出很好的抑制效果，有些已被批准用于某些癌症的治疗[79]。因此利用免疫检查点抑制剂阻断负免疫调节物对T细胞的免疫应答抑制，能有效提高T细胞免疫功能的效应。随着基因编辑技术的发展以及广泛应用，研究人员通过CRISPR-Cas9基因编辑技术靶向的去除参与免疫负调节的基因，来增强T细胞的免疫应答，有效地提高了T细胞治疗的抗肿瘤作用。该技术利用电穿孔方法将Cas9和sgRNA导入T细胞，敲除PD-1基因，使其表达减少[80-81]。经过长时间的实验观察，并未发现T细胞的活性有所降低，说明了此方法的可行性。科学家运用CRISPR-Cas9基因编辑技术有效地对 CAR-T细胞进行基因编辑，得到多基因敲除 CAR-T 细胞，成功的抑制了免疫调节物对T细胞活性的影响，提高了CAR-T 细胞抗肿瘤的效果。

4.3　在 CAR-T 细胞免疫疗法中的应用

　　CAR-T细胞免疫疗法是嵌合抗原受体T细胞免疫疗法，是一种将T细胞特殊转化后能够靶向癌细胞的免疫疗法。该方法已经经过美国食品药品监督管理局的批准，开始用于白血病和淋巴瘤等的治疗[82]。T细胞通过基因编辑技术得到修饰后，可以特异性识别肿瘤细胞表面特异性受体，并增强其对肿瘤细胞的免疫防御能力[82]。CAR-T 疗法需要采集患者的T细胞进行基因修饰，使其表面形成嵌合抗原受体的特殊结构。成为 CAR-T 细胞后再输入患者体内，协助T细胞识别攻击癌细胞（图4.2）。尽管该疗法取得了成功，但由于T 细胞数量不足或者疾病进展迅速的原因，许多患者仍无法接受这种治疗。在某些情况下，由于自身的T细胞缺陷或者CAR-T细胞无法在强免疫环境中发挥最佳作用会使该疗法的免疫反应不足[83]。

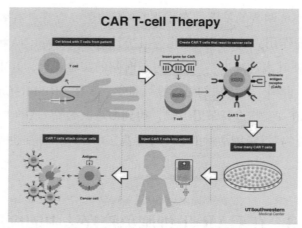

图 4.2　CAR T 细胞免疫疗法的过程 [83]

　　研究人员利用CRISPR-Cas9技术克服了这些局限性，并增强了基于CAR疗法的效应和可用性。科学家们在对正常的免疫T细胞进行引入CAR序列时，去除T细胞内源性。α β T细胞受体基因（TCRs）和人白细胞抗原Ⅰ（human leukocyte antigen Ⅰ，HLA-Ⅰ）类编码基因，防止用于不同患者时产生抗宿主反应。同时，还可以通过CRISPR-Cas9使编码信号分子的基因或T细胞抑制性受体的基因（例如PD-1）失活来提高CAR-T细胞的功能。虽然CAR-T细胞疗法的抗肿瘤疗效甚好，但是该疗法只能够特异性识别肿瘤细胞表面受体，而肿瘤特异性T细胞受体能够通过基因修饰，表达特异性受体，识别肿瘤细胞表面经Ⅰ类主要组织相容性抗原呈递的抗原肽，从而识别胞内特异性分子[84]。然而，受体T细胞的内源性TCR与修饰后的TCR可能不相容，并产生竞争反应，因此研究人员使用CRISPR-Cas9基因编辑技术干扰TCR、HLA-Ⅰ类分子和PD-1基因的表达，构建了通用的CAR-T细胞（图4.3），使其降低竞争反应，减少对宿主的损害，在抗肿瘤治疗中发挥了必不可少的作用，使该免疫疗法的作用得到大幅度的优化[85]。虽然CRISPR-Cas9基因编辑在CAR-T细胞免疫疗法中起到了优化的作用，但也存在两个限制性因素：一是通过CRISPR技术改造T细胞的方法不能使普通细胞正常增殖，限制了细胞培养和富集过程。而对于其体内导入方法，非整合转染方法虽安全但效率低，整合转染的方法效率较高，但其安全性不能保证。二是 CRISPR编辑系统存在脱靶现象，一旦发生脱靶，将导致非靶向基因的改变或调控元件的破坏，造成无法挽回的后果[86]。因此，如何避免这两个限制性因素成为未来的主要研究方向。

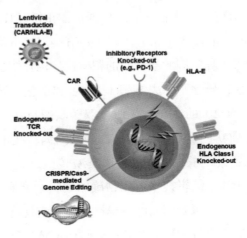

图 4.3　通过 CRISPR-Cas9 构建的通用的 CAR-T 细胞

此图片引用自参考文献[85]。

4.4　在抗体靶向疗法中的应用

肿瘤细胞表面表达了不同的抗原，但大部分都是与正常细胞不同的抗原，这一特性成为抗肿瘤研究的方向。科研人员通过构建单克隆抗体靶向识别并结合肿瘤细胞表面的特异抗原，使肿瘤细胞凋亡而达到抗肿瘤的效果。目前，研发出来的抗体类药物有很多种，如抗HER2抗体、抗CD20 抗体、抗VEGF 抗体等。CRISPR-Cas9基因编辑技术可以用来鉴别肿瘤细胞表面潜在的特异性抗原，使抗体靶向疗法发挥更好的作用。加拿大多伦多大学（University of Toronto）的Stéphane Angers研究团队利用 CRISPR-Cas9技术在具有 RNF43突变的胰腺导管肿瘤细胞之间进行全基因组筛查，发现FZD5受体在胰腺肿瘤细胞的生长中起着不可或缺的作用。与FZD5特异性结合的抗体能够显著的抑制荷瘤小鼠中癌细胞的增殖，表明 FDZ5可以作为免疫治疗药物研究的新方向[87]。

CRISPR–Cas9技术不仅在探索肿瘤细胞表面潜在抗原的靶向位点中发挥重要作用，同时也可用在抗体的制备上。根据抗体重链（H链）C区氨基酸的不同，抗体可分为 IgG、IgA、IgM、IgD 和 IgE 五类。这五类抗体在理化性质和生理功能方面存在着差异，因此在肿瘤的靶向抗体治疗中也具有不同的作用。Ig基因可以在B 细胞特异性胞苷去氨酶（AID）和细胞特异性酶，如重组激活基因蛋白1/2（RAG 1/2）的参与下使DNA双链断裂重连，实现抗体类别的转换。科学家们已经成功的运用CRISPR–Cas9基因编辑技术通过编辑人类和小鼠体内Ig基因实现了IgM–IgG–IgA的抗体类型转换，来发挥不同的抗体反应[88-89]。CRISPR–Cas9基因编辑技术可以精确的编辑杂交瘤细胞或B细胞免疫球蛋白重链恒定区的基因，得到所需的特异性抗体，实现抗肿瘤的作用。

在抗体中存在着一个标志性的片段——抗体的抗原结合片段（Fab）。Fab片段的分子量小，更容易进入肿瘤细胞，在抗肿瘤治疗中被重点关注和广泛应用。为了应用抗体Fab片段达到更高效的抗肿瘤效果，研究人员利用CRISPR–Cas9 技术删除小鼠杂交瘤细胞的Fc段的基因，获得了只分泌抗体Fab片段的杂交瘤细胞。利用CRISPR–Cas9基因编辑技术获得抗体Fab片段的方法操作简单高效，能够提高治疗效率，若与其他药物配合进入肿瘤细胞，可以达到更好的抗肿瘤治疗效果。

5　CRISPR-Cas9系统在其他医学领域的研究进展

　　除了第四章节提到的CRISPR-Cas9基因编辑技术在抗肿瘤免疫治疗中的应用，它也在其他医学领域的研究中发挥着优势，例如在构建肿瘤疾病模型中的应用，在单基因或多基因遗传病治疗方面的应用，以及在病毒性疾病治疗中的应用等。

5.1　构建肿瘤疾病模型

　　在肿瘤研究中，体细胞的遗传缺陷与病因和病理表型密切相关。随着抗肿瘤治疗方法的研究，研究人员研发了多种治疗方法，如肿瘤基因编辑，药物靶向治疗以及肿瘤耐药性的研究等，要达到临床应用则需要大量的实验验证，所以建立肿瘤疾病细胞模型成为抗肿瘤治疗必不可少的一步，CRISPR-Cas9系统则被广泛应用于建立细胞水平的肿瘤模型中。目前肺癌细胞系、乳腺癌细胞系和急性髓细胞性白血病细胞等已应用CRISPR-Cas9系统来构建肿瘤细胞模型。在建立乳腺癌细胞株模型方面，荷兰癌症研究所（The Netherlands Cancer Institute）的Stefano Annunziat等研究人员建立CRISPR-Cas9介导的乳腺癌细胞株模型，发现了一种新的HER2基因靶向抗肿瘤机制。目前治疗乳腺癌的方法主要是临床药物曲妥珠单抗，而HER2基因靶向抗肿瘤机制可以替代临床药物曲妥珠单抗，成为一种新的治疗手段[90-91]。在急性髓系白血病细胞靶向治疗方面，哈佛医学院的Takuji Yamauchi 等研究人员为了探寻急性髓系白血病（acute myeloid leukemia，AML）治疗的新靶向位点，首先对AML细胞系进行全基因组CRISPR-Cas9筛选，随后在宿主体内进行第二次筛选。他们研究确认了mRNA脱盖酶清除剂（decapping enzyme scavenger，DCPS）可诱导mRNA前体剪切错误而表现出抗白血病特性，并确定DCPS可以靶向治疗AML治疗[92]。中国蚌埠医学院Xiaojing Wang等研究人员利用 CRISPR-Cas9 建立了KRAS-突变体肺腺癌（lung adenocarcinomas，LUAD）的小鼠模型，评估了Nf1 基因缺失对 LUAD 发展的影响[93]。美国得克萨斯大学安德森癌症中心（MD Anderson Cancer Center，University of Texas）的Noboru Ideno实验室利用 CRISPR-Cas9 介导的体细胞重组构建了小鼠模型用于研究胰腺癌的治疗[94]。除肿瘤模型的建立，基于CRISPR-Cas9系统的小鼠模型还应用于其他疾病模型应用，如帕金森病、阿兹海默病等[95-96]。为了建立更接近人类生理结构的疾病模型，更好地进行药理研究和医学治疗，通过CRISPR-Cas9基因编辑系统构建的模型开始多样化，利用猪、猴或者大鼠等动物构建了多种疾病模型[102]。

5.2　治疗单基因及多基因遗传性疾病

基因疗法是指通过一些技术来改变患者体内的遗传物质，将正常的基因或者有治疗作用的基因导入到患者体内从而实现治疗的作用，分为体内治疗和体外治疗两部分。体内疗法是指将正常基因或者治疗基因导入到患者体内，体外疗法是指将患者的靶细胞取出体外，在体外进行修复扩增等处理后再次输入到患者的体内。由于CRISPR-Cas9基因编辑技术的高效性和灵活性，在基因治疗方面收到了研究人员的追捧。最近的临床试验表明，基因疗法在治疗遗传性疾病方面取得了成功。在单基因隐形连锁遗传疾病中具有代表性的是血友病，血友病的主要原因是FIX基因发生了基因突变，导致蛋白质功能减弱和血液凝固功能异常。美国华盛顿大学医学院（Washington University School of

Medicine）的Calvin Stephens 等构建了以腺病毒作为载体的研究，以幼年HB小鼠作为模型，通过CRISPR-Cas9 介导的基因编辑技术对腺病毒的基因进行了纠正，最终增强了*FIX*基因表达活性及表型矫正[97]。CRISPR-Cas9系统还可以对等位基因进行选择性编辑，通过这种方法可以为治疗多种神经退行性疾病提供重要的帮助。具有代表性的神经退行性疾病是亨廷顿舞蹈病（Huntington's disease，HD），是一种由于功能获得性胞嘧啶-腺嘌呤-鸟嘌呤（CAG）基因扩增突变引起的单基因显性遗传的神经退行性疾病。以对突变基因的处理为基础研究方向，美国马萨诸塞州综合医院（Massachusetts General Hospital）的Jun Wan Shin 等提出了一种利用CRISPR-Cas9基因编辑技术定位处理基因片段的方法，通过 CRISPR-Cas9基因编辑技术使突变的等位基因失活，敲除CAG基因的突变片段[98]。该方法使突变的等位基因完全失去活性而不影响正常等位基因的活性。2019年，*Nature Neuroscience*杂志发表了一项关于阿尔兹海默病的研究进展，该研究通过一种CRISPR-Cas9-纳米复合物，成功在体内神经元中编辑了*Bace1*基因，减轻了阿尔茨海默病小鼠模型的β淀粉样蛋白（Aβ）相关病理和认知缺陷。使用非病毒载体的Cas9-纳米复合物进行体内基因编辑的研究拓宽了CRISPR-Cas9系统在神经退行性疾病中的潜在应用。[124]美国中央密歇根大学（Central Michigan University）的Gary Dunbar实验室证实 CRISPR-Cas9 系统可以在 HD 的体外模型中诱导插入或缺失突变，减少线粒体生物标志物，在这种技术应用于临床之前，研究人员还需要进一步证明该策略的安全性和有效性[99]。CRISPR-Cas9 系统不只在单基因遗传疾病治疗中发挥了重要作用，在治疗多基因遗传病中也被广泛应用。CRISPR-Cas9系统的优势在于可通过设计多种sgRNA序列实现多个靶向位点的基因编辑，该基因编辑系统已经在阿尔茨海默病、肿瘤等多种多基因疾病的治疗中做出了贡献。

5.3　在病毒性疾病上的治疗应用

近年来，病毒引起的疾病极大地威胁着人类的生命，由于病毒的高突变率和较长的潜伏期，给治疗造成了极大地困扰，在人类体内潜伏的病毒几乎不可能被完全消除。经过科学家们不断地研究探寻，从细菌和古细菌对病毒或噬菌体的免疫防御机制中找到了灵感，使得研究人员开始从基因的角度出发寻找治疗病毒性疾病的方法。

目前，常用的抗病毒药物的作用机制主要是阻断病毒的复制周期，比如阻断病毒进入宿主细胞或是阻碍病毒的基因组复制等，但抗病毒药物只能在病毒进入复制周期时起到作用，却无法消除潜伏期病毒。因此，找到既可以阻断病毒的复制周期，又可以消除潜伏期病毒的方法成为研究人员在抗病毒治疗方面主要的研究方向。研究人员借助CRISPR-Cas系统对病毒基因组的靶向编辑，可以达到抗病毒治疗效果。2016年，荷兰乌得勒支大学医学中心（University Medical Center Utrecht）的Ferdy R. van Diemen等利用 CRISPR-Cas9技术来处理疱疹病毒，目的是抑制疱疹病毒在潜伏感染和裂解感染模型中的复制[100]。这项研究显示，利用 CRISPR-Cas9技术能够抑制三种疱疹病毒：EBV、HSV和HCMV。2018年，日本的神户大学医学研究科（Kobe University Graduate School of Medicine）的Youdiil Ophinni等研究人员设计了RNA 引导的CRISPR-Cas9靶向HIV-1调节基因tat和rev，并选择了基于六种主要HIV-1 亚型的特异性和序列保守性的 gRNA。然后在持续和潜伏的HIV-1 感染的 T 细胞系中进行了测试，结果显示 CRISPR-Cas9在持续和潜伏感染的患者 CD4和T 细胞系中能够成功抑制 HIV-1复制[101]。虽然CRISPR-Cas9系统应用于病毒性疾病治疗的方法为治疗潜伏性的病毒提供了治疗发展的方向和思路，然而对于许多具有持续性、高复发性、潜伏期长或是高度流行的病毒仍然缺乏有效的治疗方案，病毒治疗领域仍有许多未被攻克的领域，但CRISPR-Cas9系统在病毒性疾病治疗上具有很大的潜力。

6　CRISPR-Cas9存在的问题及技术改进的方法

　　尽管CRISPR-Cas9系统作为基因编辑的工具在人类遗传病基因治疗领域展现了广阔的应用前景，也有临床上的成功案例，如针对单基因遗传病，各种癌症，艾滋病等疾病进行的基因治疗，但也暴露了一定的缺陷和局限性，例如脱靶效应，传递系统的有效性和安全性，免疫排斥反应，理论争论等。

6.1　脱靶现象

　　脱靶效应（off-target effects）是因为Cas9具有切割碱基不完全配对的靶向位点的能力而引发的结果[103]。Cas9核酸酶的这种能力是在细菌和噬菌体的相互斗争进化中获得的。单链DNA或RNA病毒的遗传序列会发生突变以逃避Cas蛋白的剪切，而细菌的Cas蛋白则能够容纳低碱基错配率而进行靶向切割[104]。Cas9核酸酶对脱靶DNA的剪切是CRISPR-Cas9作为基因编辑技术的一个重要的挑战，限制了CRISPR系统在生物体内的应用。CRISPR-Cas9 基因编辑系统的特异性主要依靠sgRNA的识别序列，并与目标序列进行特异性结合。由于生物基因组序列复杂，sgRNA可能无法准确地识别靶向序列，或与其他相似序列结合造成错误剪切，导致非预期的基因突变。sgRNA在非靶位点形成局部错配的原因有两种：一是因为sgRNA与非靶向序列的DNA长度相等，但存在碱基错配；二是sgRNA与非靶向序列长度不等，通过形成DNA或RNA凸起来完成配对

（图6.1）[106]。另外，CRISPR-Cas9基因编辑系统识别标准的PAM序列，但也会识别到设计靶向序列时所忽略的非标准PAM序列，从而产生脱靶效应。

脱靶效应导致的非靶向位点突变会导致基因不能正常表达，影响其蛋白功能，为生物个体造成不可逆的损伤。早期研究利用 CRISPR-Cas9 对斑马鱼基因组进行编辑时发现，脱靶效应会影响遗传物质，并遗传给子代[105]。在癌症治疗中，脱靶效应还存在激活致癌因子，抑制抑癌基因表达的风险。为了更好地应用CRISPR-Cas9基因编辑系统，科学家们不断追寻降低脱靶效应的方法，随着基因测序技术及体外研究脱靶位点的生物化学方法的迅速发展，科学家们通过以下几种方法来降低脱靶效应，促进CRISPR-Cas9基因编辑系统更简便、更高效的应用。

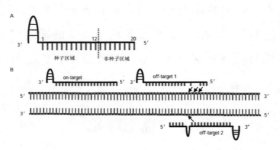

图 6.1　sgRNA 的错误配对引发的脱靶效应[106]

A：sgRNA识别目标序列依赖20个碱基，1—12碱基区域为种子区域，决定了sgRNA的识别能力，13—20号碱基为非种子区域。B：由于基因组DNA的复杂性，sgRNA不仅可与目标序列结合；也可能与非目标序列结合，激活Cas9切割活性，从而切割非目标序列，产生脱靶。off-target l是sgRNA与DNA序列在非种子区域出现3个碱基错配，of-target 2 是sgRNA与DNA序列之间存在单个凸起碱基的错配。（图中箭头所指为sgRNA与DNA错配的碱基）

6.1.1　设计高效特异性 sgRNA

引起CRISPR-Cas9基因编辑系统脱靶效应的主要原因是sgRNA无法准确地识别靶向序列引起的。因此，提高sgRNA的特异性是降低脱靶效应的一种有效方法。

sgRNA中，靠近PAM的1—12bp的碱基对称区是一段重要的区域，称为种子区域，决定了sgRNA的识别能力，而其他的序列决定了是否会产生脱靶效应。经过研究发现，碱基对称区的GC含量会影响sgRNA靶向识别效率，设计sgRNA时选择GC含量较高的序列可以降低或避免脱靶效应。设计高效特异性sgRNA可以遵循以下几点：（1）sgRNA的长度应为20 nt左右；（2）sgRNA序列的碱基组成以GC%含量40%~60%为最佳，sgRNA种子区域序列尽量避免以4个以上的T碱基结尾；（3）sgRNA的种子序列与非靶向位点的匹配数尽可能低；（4）如果构建U6或T7启动子驱动sgRNA的表达载体，需考虑sgRNA的5′碱基为G或GG，以提高其转录效率；（5）对于sgRNA靶向基因的结合位置，如需造成基因移码突变，需尽量靠近基因编码区的ATG下游，最好位于第一或第二外显子；（6）检查sgRNA靶向结合位点基因组序列是否存在SNPs或者InDels；（7）如采用Cas9n，设计paired-sgRNA需考虑成对sgRNA的间距；（8）全基因脱靶效应分析，需考虑脱靶位点最大允许的错配碱基数，建议最少5个碱基。重点考察种子序列和非种子序列碱基错配数，以及脱靶位点是否位于基因编码区等，另外还可考察是否存在碱基插入或缺失的脱靶位点[106–110]。

6.1.2 调节 Cas9-sgRNA 的浓度

在寻找降低脱靶效应的方法研究中发现，降低Cas9-sgRNA的浓度可以降低脱靶效应，研究人员发现高浓度的Cas9-sgRNA复合物有更大的概率结合非靶向序列，导致脱靶效应。Cas9在细胞中持续表达也会增加脱靶效应发生的概率，因此减低Cas9的活性也可以作为降低脱靶效应风险的方法，使用Cas9蛋白的封闭抗体或者Cas9蛋白抑制剂可以降低其在细胞中的表达[110]。虽然降低Cas9蛋白的活性或者降低Cas9-sgRNA的浓度可以降低脱靶效应的发生概率，但也会影响其正常的生理功能，降低基因组编辑能力。研究发现，当gRNA：Cas9比值为2：1或者3：1时，可以提高靶向序列的识别，降低脱靶效应[123]。

6.1.3   递送载体的选择

如何将CRISPR-Cas9编辑工具安全有效地在体内传递到靶细胞，是能否在临床上快速广泛利用的一大挑战。目前有三种传递Cas9-sgRNA的形式，分别是以质粒DNA、蛋白质或mRNA的行式传递到靶细胞中。病毒载体具有较高的编辑效率和插入突变，不能降低脱靶效应，常用的病毒载体AAV（adeno-associated virus）的最大插入承载量是4.7kb，因此无法用于插入较大的基因[111]。最合适的载体传递方式是利用不需要转录的mRNA或蛋白质形式的非病毒体内递送。通过传递纯化的Cas9-sgRNA核糖核蛋白（ribonucleoproteins，RNPs）可以更好地控制CRISPR的活性，提高编辑效率，降低脱靶效应[112]。与病毒载体相比，非病毒载体传递在临床上更具有优势，例如可以更精准的控制给药时间，减少核酸酶的长期表达，降低脱靶风险和潜在的副作用[113]。

6.1.4   Cas9 核酸酶的改造

Cas9蛋白具有两个核酸内切酶结构域，分别对DNA的两条链进行剪切，产生双链DNA的断裂。张锋实验室的研究人员构建了一种突变型Cas9蛋白，称为Cas9n，它其中的一个核酸内切酶结构域失活，只能剪切与sgRNA互补的链。因而需要两条方向相反的sgRNA分别引导Cas9n蛋白来产生双链DNA的断裂，而且产生黏性末端[114]。当一条sgRNA发生错配时，还不足以产生脱靶效应，极大地降低了脱靶效应的发生。这种方法不会太大的影响正常基因的生理功能，在人类、动植物等生物中均适用。

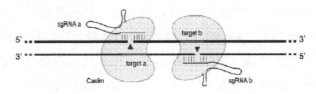

图 6.2　使用两对 sgRNA 引导的 Cas9n 进行 DNA 双链的剪切[107]

美国马萨诸塞州综合医院（Massachusetts General Hospital）的Shengdar Q

Tsai等研究人员构建了FokⅠ-dCas9复合体进行靶向位点的单链DNA切割。二聚体RNA引导的FokⅠ核酸酶（RNA-guided FokⅠnucleases，RFNs）是可以识别扩展序列并在人类细胞中高效编辑的内源基因。FokⅠ核酸酶与构建的失活Cas9（dCas9）形成融合体，通过两个不同的sgRNA引导两个FokⅠ-dCas9融合蛋白在靶向位点，以促进FokⅠ二聚化和DNA的剪切（图6.3）[115]。利用这一融合蛋白可以提高基因编辑的效率，降低脱靶效应。

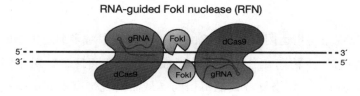

图 6.3　Fok Ⅰ-dCas9 复合体切割双链 DNA[115]

6.2　修复精准度低且错误率高

通过CRISPR-Cas9基因编辑将靶向双链DNA基因切断后，断裂处进行自我修复的主要方式是非同源末端连接（non-homologous End Joining，NHEJ），这种修复方式是通过DNA连接酶将DSBs末端直接链接的一种修复过程，不依赖于同源DNA序列，往往会引起基因的插入或删除，引发基因突变和基因功能丧失[77, 120]。在靶向位点准确的插入目标序列的修复方式，即同源修复（homology directed repair，HDR）方式所占比例常不足10%[116-117]。更好地实现CRISPR-Cas9系统的精确编辑和广泛应用，降低其修复错误率成为需要解决的问题。研究发现，可以通过抑制NHEJ修复，增加HDR的概率。HDR修复方式只有当细胞核内存在与断口DNA同源的DNA片段时才会发生。修复主要发生在细胞的S期和G2期，因此当被编辑的细胞处于G2/M期时发生同源重组的概率会大幅提高。美国休斯敦贝勒医学院（Baylor College of Medicine）的Diane Yang等研究人员通过实验证明在G2/M时期增加目标基因的编辑，可以使正确的靶向位点修复提高3～6倍[118]。此外，研究人员发现对sgRNA进行化学修饰也能达到提高HDR修复比例的效果[119]。HDR修复虽然过程复杂，但结果精确，可以通过增强HDR修复方式来提高精确基因编辑的效率。

6.3 马赛克现象（Mosacism）

马赛克现象是指运用CRISPR-Cas9基因编辑技术对多细胞生物的受精卵进行基因编辑时，受精卵在分裂阶段分裂成不同的卵裂球，针对不同的卵裂球Cas9 蛋白编辑能力和修复方式也不相同，从而出现带有不同编辑类型的细胞嵌合体，或是有些卵裂球经过了基因编辑，而有些卵裂球未被基因编辑，从而出现同时带有编辑细胞与未编辑细胞的嵌合个体，这是一个临床应用上的问题[121]。该现象出现在胚胎基因编辑领域，随着基因技术的广泛应用，研究人员希望通过基因编辑技术在胚胎早期发育时修复其突变的基因，达到治疗基因型疾病的目的。但将Cas9和 sgRNA 导入受精卵中发现了马赛克现象。研究分析推断，马赛克现象出现是由于从单细胞受精卵形成到细胞开始复制的时间较短，而Cas9基因翻译成蛋白质的时间长，错过了在单细胞时的编辑。为了避免这一现象，需要限制Cas9蛋白只在单细胞受精卵时期发挥编辑作用。日本大阪大学（Osaka University）的Masakazu Hashimoto等研究人员用电穿孔法将Cas9和sgRNA导入小鼠体外受精卵中，在小鼠受精卵首次复制之前完成基因编辑，没有检测到马赛克现象[122]。但在人体受精卵中规避这一现象还需要进一步的研究。

7　基于CRISPR-Cas9系统的突变型 RAS 肿瘤治疗新思路和研究方法

　　已开发的常用CRISPR-Cas9系统由两部分组成：引导RNA（gRNA，由crRNA和tracrRNA嵌合而成）和核酸内切酶（Cas9）。gRNA可以引导Cas9蛋白结合到基因组靶基因处，行使核酸内切酶功能切割靶基因双链DNA，利用细胞的非同源末端连接或同源重组修复机制对断裂的DNA进行插入缺失、修复或者替换，实现高效基因编辑。Cas9的核酸内切酶活性取决于RuvC-like和HNH这两个结构域，分别负责切割DNA的两条链。当这两个结构域同时被人工点突变（D10A和H840A）后，会造成Cas9丧失核酸内切酶活性成为dead Cas9（dCas9），但dCas9仍然可以在gRNA的引导下与基因组中特定的DNA序列相结合。当dCas9蛋白与转录激活因子或阻遏蛋白融合时，可以成为转录调控因子，调节基因的表达。

　　基于以上原理，我们针对含有突变型KRAS的肿瘤细胞设计了一种新颖的核酸蛋白复合物（dCas9-HDAC1/sgRNA$_{KRAS}$），目标是在不改变基因组DNA遗传信息的前提下，通过表观基因组编辑抑制K-Ras突变体蛋白的表达。此核酸蛋白复合物主要由以下两部分组成：dCas9和组蛋白去乙酰基酶1（HDAC1）构成的融合蛋白——dCas9-HDAC1，包含有与KRAS启动子区结合的由crRNA序列和tracrRNA序列构建的sgRNA$_{KRAS}$。我们的策略是：在sgRNA$_{KRAS}$的引导下，融合蛋白dCas9-HDAC1与KRAS启动子区相结合，而组蛋白去乙酰基化是表观遗传领域抑制基因表达的一个标志[125]，HDAC1可以使KRAS启动子区核心组蛋白N端部分的赖氨酸残基去乙酰基化后，与带负电荷的DNA结合变得紧密，染色质致密卷曲，从而达到抑制KRAS的转录表达的目的（图7.1）。

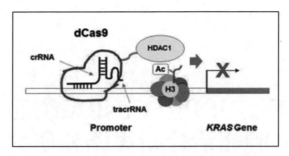

图 7.1　dCas9-HDAC1-sgRNA$_{KRAS}$ 系统抑制 *KRAS* 基因表达原理图

7.1　靶向突变型 KRAS 核酸蛋白复合物功能的初步验证

　　在前期工作中我们构建了融合基因dCas9-HDAC1的真核表达载体pcDNA3.1-dCas9-HDAC1，同时针对*KRAS*基因启动子的不同区域设计了三种不同的crRNA，范围覆盖了KRAS启动区的1 500bp的碱基序列（图7.2A）。在体外与tracrRNA形成三种不同的二聚体gRNA$_{KRAS}$，利用转染技术将pcDNA3.1-dCas9-HDAC1和gRNA$_{KRAS}$转入结肠癌细胞株HCT-116（含G13D KRAS点突变）中，Western Blot结果表明含有crRNA1和crRNA2的gRNA$_{KRAS}$与dCas9-HDAC1联合可使得K-ras蛋白表达降低，效果最为显著（图7.2B）。同理，我们发现此体系在NCI-H358（肺癌，G12C KRAS点突变）和Capan-1（胰腺癌，G12V KRAS点突变）中同样有效（图7.2C和图7.2D）。

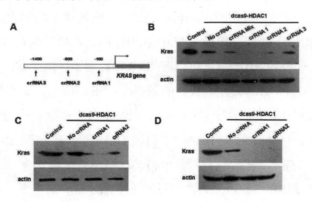

图 7.2　针对 *KRAS* 基因启动子的不同区域设计的三种 crRNA

A—KRAS 启动子区 crRNA 的位置以及覆盖的范围；B—Western Blot 结果表明 dCas9-HDAC1/gRNA$_{KRAS}$系统在结肠癌抑制 K-ras 表达；C—Western Blot 结果表明 dCas9-HDAC1/gRNA$_{KRAS}$系统在肺癌抑制 K-ras 表达；D—Western Blot 结果表明 dCas9-HDAC1/gRNA$_{KRAS}$系统在胰腺癌抑制 K-ras 表达。

我们还发现应用了此体系降低 K-ras 蛋白表达后，显著抑制了这三种肿瘤细胞株的增殖（图7.3），同时增加了它们的凋亡比率（图7.4）。前期的实验结果初步证明了我们设计的 dCas9-HDAC1/sgRNA$_{KRAS}$体系的有效性。

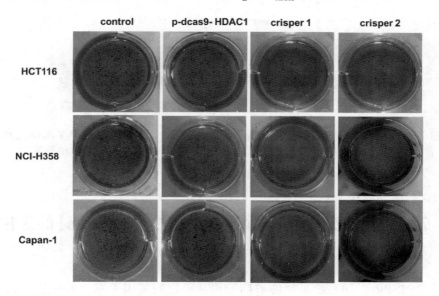

图 7.3　克隆形成实验结果表明 dCas9-HDAC/gRNA$_{KRAS}$ 系统抑制了结肠癌细胞 HCT-116、肺癌细胞 NCI-H358、胰腺癌细胞 Capan-1 的细胞增殖

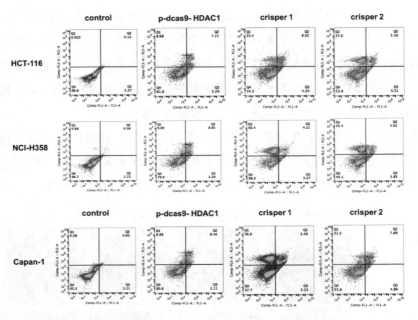

图 7.4　流式细胞术结果表明 dCas9–HDAC1/gRNA$_{KRAS}$ 系统诱导了结肠癌细胞 HCT–116、肺癌细胞 NCI–H358 和胰腺癌细胞 Capan–1 的细胞凋亡

7.2　靶向突变型 KRAS 核酸蛋白复合物设计的优化

　　CRISPR/Cas9系统虽然能够高效快速地进行基因编辑，但该技术的重要缺点是"脱靶效应"，即设计的gRNA会与非靶点DNA序列错配，引入非预期的基因突变。这阻碍了该项技术在临床的应用，但随着研究的不断发展，目前研究人员也设计很多对策来解决此问题，例如Chen JS团队在*Nature*上发表课题组的研究成果，他们对Cas9进行了点突变改造成超精确Cas9蛋白（HypaCas9），极大程度上降低了脱靶效应；用单链引导RNA（sgRNA）代替crRNA和tracrRNA的二聚体并优化其序列[126]等。在2020年3月4日，Allergan和Editas Medicine公司在一项1/2期临床试验研究中已完成首例患者给药，使用CRISPR基因编辑手段（EDIT–101）治疗Leber先天性黑蒙10型患者，这是世界

上首个患者体内给药的CRISPR基因编辑疗法，表现出CRISPR技术在安全性方面的又一个进步。因此，我们拟采用相似的策略对pcDNA3.1-dCas9-HDAC1进行点突变改造后，制备Hypa-dCas9-HDAC1融合蛋白，同时根据我们实验验证过的crRNA设计，并优化相应sgRNA以降低本系统的脱靶效应。

　　本项目之所以选用dCas9-HDAC1蛋白代替真核表达载体，是由于该蛋白是非持续表达且可降解，因此，可以显著降低脱靶效应。除此之外，还有很多其他优点：如因为没引入外源DNA序列而可以避免非预期的基因片段插入；不需转录表达与降解质粒，无免疫反应干扰；有研究表明Cas9蛋白与sgRNA结合效率更高、更稳定，可以提高编辑效率等。

8　总结与展望

　　CRISPR-Cas系统作为在细菌和古细菌中的一种获得性免疫防御系统，从发现并不断地探索研究到现在的广泛应用，这一系列发展过程离不开研究人员的辛勤探索。人类的研究逐渐深入到了基因研究层面，如今基因疗法已经成为治疗疾病的新兴手段。经过对该系统不断地发现探索和完善，CRISPR-Cas9 系统成为一种新型的基因编辑技术。因为CRISPR-Cas9 系统可以定向编辑，操作简单，成本低且效率高，适用于绝大多数的生物体等优点，被称为最具有发展前景的基因编辑技术，在临床试验中得到了广泛应用。CRISPR-Cas9基因编辑系统被应用在抗肿瘤和抗病毒治疗，以及多种单基因或多基因遗传病的治疗。虽然CRISPR-Cas9基因编辑系统在医学研究和临床试验上有很多的成果，但该系统还存在着一定的缺陷，如脱靶效应、马赛克现象、精确修复率低等，尤其是脱靶效应，可能会造成正常基因突变，蛋白功能丧失，或引发其他的遗传性疾病。如今针对脱靶效应已经研究出了多种规避方法，但其处理步骤烦琐、难操作，降低了该系统的利用效率，因此仍需探索出高效、简便的降低脱靶效应的方法。对于马赛克现象，目前还未探索出规避的方法，需要不断地研究和试验。然而可以肯定的是，随着科研人员的投入和研究技术的发展，CRISPR-Cas系统会不断有新发现，作为基因编辑技术也会向着精准、简单和高效等方面不断进步。相信在不断地探索和发展中，CRISPR-Cas基因编辑系统会为生物领域、医学领域以及临床治疗等方面提供更多的资源和应用，成为最具有发展前景的一项基因编辑技术。

参考文献

[1] BARRANGOU, RODOTPHE, FREMAUX, et al. CRISPR provides acquired resistance against viruses in prokaryotes[J]. Science, 2007, 315 (5819): 1709–1712.

[2] BOLOTIN A, QUINQUIS B, SOROKIN A, et al. Clustered regularly interspaced short palindrome repeats (CRISPRs) have spacers of extrachromosomal origin[J]. Microbiology, 2005, 151 (8): 2551–2561.

[3] RANDALL J. PLATT. CRISPR–Cas9 Knockin Mice for Genome Editing and Cancer Modeling[J]. Cell, 2014, 159 (2): 440–455.

[4] ISHINO Y, SHINAGAWA H, MAKINO K, et al. Nucleotide sequence of the iap gene, responsible for alkaline phosphatase isozyme conversion in Escherichia coli, and identification of the gene product[J]. Journal of bacteriology, 1987, 169 (12): 5429–5433.

[5] GROENEN P M A, BUNSCHOTEN A E, SOOLINGEN D V, et al. Nature of DNA polymorphism in the direct repeat cluster of mycobacterium tuberculosis; application for strain differentiation by a novel typing method[J]. Molecular Microbiology, 2010, 10 (5): 1057–1065.

[6] MOJICA F J M, FERRER C, JUEZ G, et al. Long stretches of short tandem repeats are present in the largest replicons of the Archaea Haloferax mediterranei and Haloferax volcanii and could be involved in replicon partitioning[J]. Molecular Microbiology, 2010, 17 (1): 85–93.

[7] MASEPOHL B, GORLITZ K, BOHME H, et al. Long tandemly repeated repetitive (LTRR) sequences in the filamentous cyanobacterium Anabaena sp. PCC 7120[J]. Biochimica et Biophysica Acta (BBA) – Gene Structure and Expression, 1996, 1307 (1): 26–30.

[8] HOE N, NAKASHIMA K, GRIGSBY D, et al. Rapid molecular genetic subtyping of serotype M1 group A Streptococcus strains[J]. Emerging Infectious Diseases, 1999, 5 (2): 254–263.

[9] GROENEN P M A, BUNSCHTEN A E, SOOLINGEN D V, et, al. CRISPR/Cas, the

immune system of bacteria and archaea[J]. Science, 2010, 327（5962）: 167-170.

[10] Terns M P, Terns R M. CRISPR-based adaptive immune systems[J]. Current Opinion in Microbiology, 2011, 14（3）: 321-327.

[11] MOJICA F J M, DIEZ-VILLASENOR C, SORIA E, et al. Biological significance of a family of regularly spaced repeats in the genomes of Archaea, Bacteria and mitochondria[J]. Molecular Microbiology, 2010, 36（1）: 244-246.

[12] JANSEN R, EMBDEN J D A V, GAASTRA W, et al. Identification of genes that are associated with DNA repeats in prokaryotes[J]. Molecular Microbiology, 2002, 43（6）: 1565-1575.

[13] Makarova K S, Aravind L, Grishin N V, et al. A DNA repair system specific for thermophilic Archaea and bacteria predicted by genomic context analysis[J]. Nucleic Acids Research, 2002, 30（2）: 482-496. .

[14] GUY C P, MAJERNÍK ALAN I, CHONG J P J, et al. A novel nuclease-ATPase（Nar71）from archaea is part of a proposed thermophilic DNA repair system[J]. Nucleic Acids Research, 2004, 32（21）: 6176-6186.

[15] MOJICA F J M, CÉSAR DÍEZ-VILLASEÑOR, JESÚS GARCÍA-MARTÍNEZ, et al. Intervening sequences of regularly spaced prokaryotic repeats derive from foreign genetic elements[J]. Journal of molecular evolution, 2005, 60（2）: 174-182.

[16] POURCEL C. CRISPR elements in Yersinia pestis acquire new repeats by preferential uptake of bacteriophage DNA, and provide additional tools for evolutionary studies[J]. Microbiology, 2005, 151（3）: 653-663.

[17] TANG T H, BACHELLERIE J P, ROZHDESTVENSKY T, et al. Identification of 86 candidates for small non-messenger RNAs from the archaeon Archaeoglobus fulgidus[J]. Proceedings of the National Academy of Sciences of the United States of America, 2002, 99（11）: 7536-7536.

[18] HAFT D H, SELENGUT J, MONGODIN E F, et al. A Guild of 45 CRISPR-Associated（Cas）Protein Families and Multiple CRISPR/Cas Subtypes Exist in Prokaryotic Genomes[J]. Plos Computational Biology, 2005, 1（6）.

[19] MAKAROVA K S, GRISHIN N V, SHABALINA S A, et al. A putative RNA-interference-based immune system in prokaryotes: computational analysis of the predicted enzymatic machinery, functional analogies with eukaryotic RNAi, and hypothetical mechanisms of action [J]. Biology Direct, 2006, 1（1）: 7.

[20] BARRANGOU R, HORVATH P. CRISPR: New horizons in phage resistance and strain

identification[J]. Annual Review of Food Science & Technology, 2012, 3（1）: 143.

[21] STAN J J, BROUNS, MATTHIJS M, et al. Small CRISPR RNAs guide antiviral defense in prokaryotes[J]. Science, 2008, 321（5891）: 960-964.

[22] MARRAFFINI L A, SONTHEIMER E J. CRISPR interference limits horizontal gene transfer in staphylococci by targeting DNA [J]. Science, 2008, 322（5909）: 1843-1845.

[23] ANDERSSON A F, BANFIELD J F. Virus population dynamics and acquired virus resistance in natural microbial communities[J]. Science, 2008, 320（5879）: 1047-1050.

[24] MOJICA F J M, DIEZ-VILLASENOR C, GARCIA-MARTINEZ J, et al. Short motif sequences determine the targets of the prokaryotic CRISPR defence system[J]. Microbiology, 2009, 155（3）: 733-740.

[25] MARRAFFINI L A, SONTHEIMER E J. CRISPR interference limits horizontal gene transfer in staphylococci by targeting DNA[J]. Science, 2008, 322（5909）: 1843-1845.

[26] DELTCHEVA E, CHYLINSKI K, SHARMA C M, et al. CRISPR RNA maturation by trans-encoded small RNA and host factor RNase Ⅲ [J]. Nature, 2011, 471（7340）: 602-607.

[27] MAKAROVA K S, HAFT D H, BARRANGOU R, et al. Evolution and classification of the CRISPR - Cas systems[J]. Nature Reviews Microbiology, 2011, 9（6）: 467-477.

[28] JINEK, MARTIN, CHYLINSKI, et al. A Programmable Dual-RNA-Guided DNA Endonuclease in Adaptive Bacterial Immunity[J]. Science, 2012, 337（6096）: 816-821.

[29] WIEDENHEFT B, STERNBERG S H, DOUDNA J A. RNA-guided genetic silencing systems in bacteria and archaea[J]. Nature, 2012, 482（7385）: 331-338.

[30] CONG L, RAN F A, COX D, et al. Multiplex genome engineering using CRISPR/Cas systems[J]. Science, 2013, 339（6121）: 819-823

[31] FRIEDLAND A E, TZUR Y B, ESVELT K M, et al. Heritable genome editing in C. elegans via a CRISPR-Cas9 system. [J]. Nature methods, 2013, 10（8）: 741-743.

[32] Gilbert L A, MATTHEW H L, LEONARDO M, et al. CRISPR-mediated modular RNA-guided regulation of transcription in eukaryotes [J]. Cell, 2013, 154（2）: 442-451.

[33] ZETSCHE B, GOOTENBERG J, ABUDAYYEH O, et al. Cpf1 is a single RNA-guided endonuclease of a class 2 CRISPR-Cas system[J]. Cell, 2015, 163（3）: 759-771.

[34] KOMOR A C, KIM Y B, PACKER M S, et al. Programmable editing of a target base in genomic DNA without double-stranded DNA cleavage[J]. Nature, 2016, 533（7603）: 420-424.

[35] GAUDELLI N M, KOMOR A C, RESS H A, et al. Programmable base editing of A•T to G•C

in genomic DNA without DNA cleavage[J]. Nature, 2017, 551（7681）: 464–471.

[36] SHMAKOV S, ABUDAYYEH O O, MAKAROVA K S, et al. Discovery and functional characterization of diverse class 2 CRISPR–Cas systems [J]. Molecular Cell, 2015, 60（3）: 385–391.

[37] YANG H, GAO P, RAJASHANKAR K R, et al. PAM–dependent target DNA recognition and cleavage by C2c1 CRISPR–Cas endonuclease[J]. Cell, 2016, 167（7）: 1814–1828.

[38] LIU L, CHEN P, WANG M, et al. C2c1–sgRNA complex structure reveals RNA–guided DNA cleavage mechanism[J]. Molecular cell, 2016, 65（2）: 310.

[39] STRECKER J , JONES S , KOOPAL B , et al. Engineering of CRISPR–Cas12b for human genome editing[J]. Nature Communications, 2019, 10（1）: 866–869.

[40] JOSIANE E G, MARIE–ÈVE DUPUIS, MANUELA V, et al. The CRISPR/Cas bacterial immune system cleaves bacteriophage and plasmid DNA[J]. Nature, 2010, 468（7320）: 67–71.

[41] MAKAROVA K S, WOLF Y I, ALKHNBASHI O S, et al. An updated evolutionary classification of CRISPR–Cas systems[J]. Nature reviews. Microbiology, 2015, 13（11）: 722–36.

[42] GASIUNAS G, BARRANGOU R, HORVATH P, et al. Cas9–crRNA ribonucleoprotein complex mediates specific DNA cleavage for adaptive immunity in bacteria[J]. Proceedings of the National Academy of Sciences of the United States of America, 2012, 109（39）: 15539–15540.

[43] BARRANGOU R, FREMAUX C, HÉLÈNE DEVEAU, et al. CRISPR provides acquired resistance against viruses in prokaryotes[J]. Science, 2007, 315（5819）: 1709–1712.

[44] GARNEAU J E, DUPUIS J E, VILLION M, et al. The CRISPR/Cas bacterial immune system cleaves bacteriophage and plasmid DNA. [J]. Nature, 2010, 468（7320）: 67–71.

[45] SAPRANAUSKAS R, GASIUNAS G, FREMAUX C, et al. The streptococcus thermophilus CRISPR/Cas system provides immunity in escherichia coli. nucleic acids res[J]. Nucleic Acids Research, 2011, 39（21）: 9275–9282.

[46] JACKSON S A, MCKENZIE R E, FAGERLUND R D, et al. CRISPR–Cas: Adapting to change[J]. Science, 2017, 356（6333）: 5056.

[47] BARRANGOU R, HORVATH P. A decade of discovery: CRISPR functions and applications[J]. Nature Microbiology, 2017, 2（7）: 17092.

[48] JIANG F G, JENNIFER. CRISPR‐Cas9 structures and mechanisms[J]. Annual Review of Biophysics, 2017, 46（1）: 505–529.

[49] DOUDNA J A, CHARPENTIER E, et al. The new frontier of genome engineering with CRISPR-Cas9[J]. Science, 2014, 346（6213）: 1258096.

[50] STAALS R H J, JACKSON S A, BISWAS A, et al. Interference-driven spacer acquisition is dominant over naive and primed adaptation in a native CRISPR - Cas system[J]. Nature Communications, 2016, 7（1）: 12853.

[51] HELER R, SAMAI P, MODELL J W, et al. Cas9 specifies functional viral targets during CRISPR-Cas adaptation[J]. Nature, 2015, 519（7542）: 199-202.

[52] SERGEY S, EKATERINA S, EKATERINA S, et al. Pervasive generation of oppositely oriented spacers during CRISPR adaptation[J]. Nucleic acids research, 2014, 42（9）: 5907-5916.

[53] SWARTS D C, MOSTERD C, PASSEL M W J V, et al. CRISPR interference directs strand specific spacer acquisition [J]. PLOS ONE, 2012, 7（4）: 35888.

[54] CARTE J, CHRISTOPHER R T, SMITH J T, et al. The three major types of CRISPR-Cas systems function independently in CRISPR RNA biogenesis in Streptococcus thermophilus[J]. Molecular Microbiology, 2014, 93（1）: 98-112.

[55] MAKAROVA K S, ZHANG F, KOONIN E V. SnapShot: Class 1 CRISPR-Cas systems[J]. Cell, 2017, 168（5）: 946-946.

[56] MAKAROVA K S, KOONIN E V. Annotation and classification of CRISPR-Cas systems[J]. Methods Mol Biol, 2015, 1311: 47-75.

[57] MAKAROVA K S, ARAVIND L, WOLF Y I, et al. Unification of Cas protein families and a simple scenario for the origin and evolution of CRISPR-Cas systems[J]. Biology Direct, 2011, 6（1）: 38.

[58] VESTERGAARD G, GARRETT R A, SHAH S A. CRISPR adaptive immune systems of Archaea[J]. Rna Biology, 2014, 11（2）: 156-167.

[59] HELER R, SAMAI P, MODELL J W, et al. Cas9 specifies functional viral targets during CRISPR-Cas adaptation[J]. Nature, 2015, 519（7542）: 199-202.

[60] WEI Y Z, REBECCA M, MICHAEL P, et al. Cas9 function and host genome sampling in Type Ⅱ-A CRISPR - Cas adaptation[J]. Genes & Development, 2015, 29（4）, 356-361.

[61] KRZYSZTOF C, MAKAROVA K S, EMMANUELLE C, et al. Classification and evolution of type Ⅱ CRISPR-Cas systems[J]. Nucleic Acids Research, 2014（10）: 6091-6105.

[62] CHYLINSKI K, ANAÏS L R, CHARPENTIERE. The tracrRNA and Cas9 families of type Ⅱ CRISPR-Cas immunity systems[J]. RNA Biology, 2013, 10（5）: 726-737.

[63] INES F, ANAÏS L R, KRZYSZTOF C, et al. Phylogeny of Cas9 determines functional exchangeability of dual-RNA and Cas9 among orthologous type Ⅱ CRISPR-Cas systems[J]. Nucleic Acids Research, 2014, 42（4）: 2577-2590.

[64] MAKAROVA K S, WOLF Y I, KOONIN E V. Classification and nomenclature of CRISPR-Cas systems: where from here?[J]. The CRISPR Journal, 2018, 1（5）: 325-336.

[65] MAKAROVA K S, WOLF Y I, IRANZO J, et al. Evolutionary classification of CRISPR-Cas systems: a burst of class 2 and derived variants[J]. Nature Reviews Microbiology, 2019, 18（2）: 67-83.

[66] STRECKER J, JONES S, KOOPAL B, et al. Engineering of CRISPR-Cas12b for human genome editing[J]. Nature Communications, 2019, 10（1）: 212.

[67] SWARTS D C, JINEK M. Mechanistic insights into the cis- and trans-Acting DNase Activities of Cas12a[J]. Molecular Cell, 2019, 73（3）: 589-600.

[68] MEESKE A J, NAKANDAKARI-HIGA S, MARRAFFINI L A. Cas13-induced cellular dormancy prevents the rise of CRISPR-resistant bacteriophage[J]. Nature, 2019, 570（7760）: 241-245.

[69] HARRINGTON L B, BURSTEIN D, CHEN J S, et al. Programmed DNA destruction by miniature CRISPR-Cas14 enzymes[J]. Science, 2018, 362（6416）: 4294.

[70] KARVELIS T, BIGELYTE G, YOUNG J K, et al. PAM recognition by miniature CRISPR-Cas12f nucleases triggers programmable double-stranded DNA target cleavage[J]. Nucleic Acids Research, 2020, 48（9）.

[71] YAN W X, HUNNEWELL P, ALFONSE L E, et al. Functionally diverse type V CRISPR-cas systems[J]. Science, 2018, 363（6422）: 88-91.

[72] SHMAKOV S, SMARGON A, SCOTT D, et al. Diversity and evolution of class 2 CRISPR-Cas systems[J]. Nature Reviews Microbiology, 2017, 15（3）: 169-182.

[73] KOONIN E V, MAKAROVA K S. Mobile Genetic Elements and Evolution of CRISPR-Cas Systems: All the Way There and Back[J]. Genome Biology & Evolution（10）: 2812-2825.

[74] FAURE G, SHMAKOV S A, YAN W X, et al. CRISPR-Cas in mobile genetic elements: counter-defence and beyond[J]. Nature Reviews Microbiology, 2019, 17（8）: 1-13.

[75] SHMAKOV S, ABUDAYYEH O O, MAKAROVA K S, et al. Discovery and functional characterization of diverse class 2 CRISPR-Cas systems[J]. Molecular cell, 2015, 60（3）: 385-397.

[76] ABUDAYYEH O O, GOOTENBERG J S, PATRICK E, et al. RNA targeting with CRISPR-

Cas13[J]. Nature, 2017, 550（7675）: 280-284.

[77] JENKINS R W, BARBIE D A, FLAHERTY K T. Mechanisms of resistance to immune checkpoint inhibitors[J]. British Journal of Cancer, 2018, 118（1）: 9-16.

[78] DARVIN P, TOOR S M, SASIDHARAN NAIR V, et al. Immune checkpoint inhibitors: recent progress and potential biomarkers[J]. Experimental & Molecular Medicine, 2018, 50（12）: 1-11.

[79] ZINDL C L, CHAPLIN D D. Immunology. Tumor immune evasion[J]. Science, 2010, 328（5979）: 697 — 698.

[80] SU S, ZOU Z, CHEN F, et al. CRISPR-Cas9-mediated disruption of PD-1 on human T cells for adoptive cellular therapies of EBV positive gastric cancer[J]. Oncoimmunology, 2017, 6（1）: 1249558.

[81] JUNE C H, O'CONNOR R S, KAWALEKAR O U, et al. CAR T cell immunotherapy for human cancer[J]. Science, 2018, 359（6382）: 1361-1365.

[82] FRAIETTA J A, LACEY S F, ORLANDO E, et al. Determinants of response and resistance to CD19 chimeric antigen receptor (CAR) T cell therapy of chronic lymphocytic leukemia [J]. Nature Medicine, 2018, 24（5）: 563-571.

[83] JORDAN B. First use of CRISPR for gene therapy[J]. Medecine Sciences M/s, 2016, 32（11）: 1035-1037.

[84] SALAS-MCKEE J, KONG W, GLADNEY W L, et al. CRISPR/Cas9-based genome editing in the era of CAR T cell immunotherapy[J]. Human Vaccines & Immunotherapeutics, 2019, 15（5）: 1126-1132.

[85] VITA G. CAR-T Cell Therapy: From the Bench to the Bedside[J]. Cancers, 2017, 9（12）: 150.

[86] YAMAUCHI T, MASUDA T, CANVER M C, et al. Genome-wide CRISPR-Cas9 screen identifies leukemia-specific dependence on a pre-mRNA metabolic pathway regulated by DCPS[J]. Cancer Cell, 2018, 33（3）: 386-400.

[87] SÉBASTIEN ANGUILLE, SMITS E L, BRYANT C, et al. Dendritic cells as pharmacological tools for cancer immunotherapy[J]. Pharmacological Reviews, 2015, 67（4）: 731-753.

[88] 龚晨雨, 陈昭, 邵红伟, 等. CRISPR/Cas9 基因编辑技术在肿瘤免疫治疗中的应用 [J]. 中国免疫学杂志, 2018, 34（01）: 122-126.

[89] ANNUNZIATO S, KAS S M, NETHE M, et al. Modeling invasive lobular breast carcinoma by CRISPR/Cas9-mediated somatic genome editing of the mammary gland[J]. Cold Spring Harbor Laboratory Press, 2016, 30（12）: 1470-1480.

[90] SLAMON D J, LEYLAND J B, SHAK S, et al. Use of chemotherapy plus a Monoclonal antibody against HER2 for metastatic breast cancer that overexpresses HER2[J]. The New England Journal of Medicine, 2001, 344（11）: 783-792.

[91] YAMAUCHI T, MASUDA T, CANVER M C, et al. Genome-wide CRISPR-Cas9 screen identifies leukemia-specific dependence on a pre-mRNA metabolic pathway regulated by DCPS[J]. Cancer Cell, 2018, 33（3）: 386-400.

[92] WANG X, MIN S, LIU H, et al. Nf1 loss promotes Kras -driven lung adenocarcinoma and results in Psat1-mediated glutamate dependence[J]. EMBO Molecular Medicine, 2019, 11（6）: 9856.

[93] IDENO N, YAMAGUCHI H, OKUMURA T, et al. A pipeline for rapidly generating genetically engineered mouse models of pancreatic cancer using in vivo CRISPR-Cas9-mediated somatic recombination[J]. Laboratory Investigation, 2009, 99（3）: 1233-1244.

[94] JAESUK, LEE, DELGER, et al. CRISPR/Cas9 Edited sRAGE-MSCs Protect Neuronal Death in Parkinson`s Disease Model. [J]. International Journal of Stem Cells, 2019, 12（1）.

[95] HANSEUL P, JUNGJU O, GAYONG S, et al. In vivo neuronal gene editing via CRISPR‐Cas9 amphiphilic nanocomplexes alleviates deficits in mouse models of Alzheimer's disease [J]. Nature Neuroscience, 2019, 22: 524-528.

[96] STEPHENS C J, LAURON E J, KASHENTSEVA E, et al. Long-term correction of hemophilia B using adenoviral delivery of CRISPR/Cas9[J]. Journal of Controlled Release, 2019, 298: 128-141.

[97] SHIN J W, KIM K H, CHAO M J, et al. Permanent inactivation of Huntington's disease mutation by personalized allele-specific CRISPR/Cas9[J]. Human Molecular Genetics, 2016, 25（20）: 4566-4576.

[98] DUNBAR GL, KONERU S, KOLLI N, et al. Silencing of the mutant huntingtin gene through CRISPR-Cas9 improves the mitochondrial biomarkers in an in vitro model of Huntington's disease[J]. Cell Transplant, 2019, 28（4）: 460-463.

[99] DIEMEN F R V, KRUSE E M, HOOYKAAS M J G, et al. CRISPR/Cas9-mediated genome editing of herpesviruses limits productive and latent infections[J]. Plos Pathogens, 2016, 12（6）: 1005701.

[100] OPHINNI Y, INOUE M, KOTAKI T, et al. CRISPR/Cas9 system targeting regulatory genes of HIV-1 inhibits viral replication in infected T-cell cultures[J]. Scientific Reports, 2018, 8

（1）：7784.

[101] YANG L，MARC GÜELL，NIU D，et al. Genome-wide inactivation of porcine endogenous retroviruses（PERVs）[J]. Science，2015，350（6264）：1101-1104.

[102] HERAI R H. Avoiding the off-target effects of CRISPR/cas9 system is still a challenging accomplishment for genetic transformation[J]. Gene，2019，700：176-178.

[103] LI J，SUN J，GAO X，et al. Coupling ssDNA recombineering with CRISPR-Cas9 for Escherichia coli DnaG mutations[J]. Applied microbiology and biotechnology，2019，103（8）：3559-3570.

[104] HRUSCHA A，KRAWITZ P，RECHENBERG A，et al. Efficient CRISPR/Cas9 genome editing with low off-target effects in zebrafish[J]. Development，2013，140（24）：4982-4987.

[105] 袁伟曦，喻云梅，胡春财，等. CRISPR/Cas9 技术存在的问题及其改进措施的研究进展 [J]. 生物技术通报，2017，33（4）：70-77.

[106] HSU P，LANDER E，ZHANG F. Development and Applications of CRISPR-Cas9 for Genome Engineering[J]. Cell，2014，157（6）：1262-1278.

[107] PAQUET D，KWART D，CHEN A，et al. Efficient introduction of specific homozygous and heterozygous mutations using CRISPR/Cas9. J]. Nature，2016，533（7601）：125-129.

[108] CHU V T，WEBER T，WEFERS B，et al. Increasing the efficiency of homology-directed repair for CRISPR-Cas9-induced precise gene editing in mammalian cells[J]. Nature Biotechnology，2015，33（5）：543-548.

[109] ASCHENBRENNER S，KALLENBERGER S M，HOFFMANN M D，et al. Coupling Cas9 to artificial inhibitory domains enhances CRISPR-Cas9 target specificity[J]. Science Advances，2020，6（6）：eaay 0187.

[110] NASO M F，TOMKOWICZ B，PERRYIII W L，et al. Adeno-Associated Virus (AAV) as a Vector for Gene Therapy[J]. BioDrugs，2017，31（4）：317-334.

[111] KIM S，KIM D，CHO S W，et al. Highly efficient RNA-guided genome editing in human cells via delivery of purified Cas9 ribonucleoproteins[J]. Genome Research，2014，24（6）：1012-1019.

[112] YIN H，SONG C Q，DORKIN J R，et al. Therapeutic genome editing by combined viral and non-viral delivery of CRISPR system components in vivo[J]. Nature Biotechnology，2016，34（3）：328-333.

[113] RAN F A，HSU P D，CHIE Y L，et al. Double Nicking by RNA-Guided CRISPR Cas9 for

Enhanced Genome Editing Specificity[J]. Cell，2013，154（6）：1380–1389.

[114] TSAI S Q，WYVEKENS N，KHAYTER C，et al. Dimeric CRISPR RNA–guided FokI nucleases for highly specific genome editing[J]. Nature biotechnology，2014，32（6）：569–576.

[115] PAQUET D，KWART D，CHEN A，et al. Efficient introduction of specific homozygous and heterozygous mutations using CRISPR/Cas9[J]. Nature，2016，533（7601）：125–129.

[116] MIYAOKA Y，BERMAN J R，COOPER S B，et al. Systematic quantification of HDR and NHEJ reveals effects of locus，nuclease，and cell type on genome–editing[J]. Scientific Reports，2016，6：23549.

[117] YANG D，SCAVUZZO M A，CHMIELOWIEC J，et al. Enrichment of G2/M cell cycle phase in human pluripotent stem cells enhances HDR–mediated gene repair with customizable endonucleases[J]. Scientific Reports，2016，6（1）：21264.

[118] HENDEL A，BAK R O，CLARK J T，et al. Chemically modified guide RNAs enhance CRISPR–Cas genome editing in human primary cells[J]. Nature Biotechnology，2015，33（9）：985–989.

[119] YANG D，SCAVUZZO M A，CHMIELOWIEC J，et al. Enrichment of G2/M cell cycle phase in human pluripotent stem cells enhances HDR–mediated gene repair with customizable endonucleases[J]. Scientific Reports，2016，6（1）：21264.

[120] MEHRAVAR M，SHIRAZI A，NAZARI M，et al. Mosaicism in CRISPR/Cas9–mediated genome editing[J]. Developmental Biology，2019，445（2）：156–162.

[121] HASHIMOTO M，YAMASHITA Y，TAKEMOTO T. Electroporation of Cas9 protein/sgRNA into early pronuclear zygotes generates non–mosaic mutants in the mouse[J]. Developmental Biology，2016，418（1）：1–9.

[122] 郭全娟，韩秋菊，张建. Off–target Effect of CRISPR/Cas9 and Optimization[J]. 生物化学与生物物理进展，2018，45（8）：798–807.

[123] TOH T B，LIM J J，CHOW K H. Epigenetics in cancer stem cells[J]. Molecular Cancer，2017，16（1）：29.

[124] KWON D Y，ZHAO Y T，LAMONICA J M，et al. Locus–specific histone deacetylation using a synthetic CRISPR–Cas9–based HDAC[J]. Nature Communications，2017，8（1）：15315.

[125] CHEN J S，DAGDAS Y S，KLEINSTIVER B P，et al. Enhanced proofreading governs CRISPR–cas9 targeting accuracy[J]. Biophysical Journal，2018，114（3）：194.

第三部分

基因编辑传递系统及外泌体的应用

摘　要

　　基因治疗的核心是基因编辑技术。基因编辑是指对基因组特定位点进行编辑，实现定点突变、插入或敲除的一项技术。实现在真核生物尤其是哺乳动物中的精准基因编辑始于依赖核酸酶的基因编辑技术，直接插入细胞的基因通常难以表达，因此需要构建包含目标基因的载体来传递该基因。细菌质粒是一种独立于细菌拟核之外、结构简单、可自我复制的环状DNA分子，质粒通常含有一个至多个限制性酶切位点供外源DNA片段插入，是一种常用的载体。某些病毒或噬菌体衍生物也会被用作载体，因为它们可以通过感染细胞来传递遗传物质。利用质粒或病毒载体可能会存在潜在的安全问题，目前蛋白质和RNA也被研究用作载体完成目的基因的导入。携带目标基因的载体会将其整合到细胞的染色体中，抑或只将其引入到细胞核内。携带目的基因的载体种类繁多，其转运效率、靶向率、基因突变率或目的基因表达效率，以及可能存在的潜在威胁也各不相同，本章节将详细讲解基因编辑用到的不同传递系统，并重点讲解细胞内源物外泌体作为载体的研究和应用。

　　【关键词】基因编辑；递送系统；载体；质粒；病毒；脂质体；外泌体

Abstract

The core of gene therapy is the technology of gene editing. Gene editing refers to the editing of specific sites in the genome to achieve site-directed mutation, insertion, or knockout. Realizing precise gene editing in eukaryotes, especially mammals, starts with gene editing techniques that rely on nucleases. Genes directly inserted into cells are usually difficult to express. Therefore, it is necessary to construct a vector containing the target gene to deliver the gene. A bacterial plasmid is a circular DNA molecule with a simple structure and self-replicating independent of the bacterial nucleus. The plasmid usually contains one or more restriction sites for the insertion of foreign DNA fragments. It is a commonly used vector. Certain viruses or phage derivatives are also used as vectors because they can infect cells to deliver genetic material. The use of plasmids or viral vectors may have potential safety issues. At present, proteins and RNA have also been studied as vectors to complete the introduction of target genes. The vector carrying the target gene will integrate it into the chromosome of the cell, or only introduce it into the nucleus. There are many types of vectors carrying target genes, and their delivery efficiency, targeting rate, gene mutation rate or target gene expression efficiency, and possible potential threats are various. This chapter will explain in detail the different delivery systems used in gene editing with a focus on the research and application of exosomes as carriers.

[Keywords] Gene editing; delivery systems; vectors; plasmid; virus; liposome; exosome

随着科技的不断进步，我们的探索也逐渐由简入繁，由大体到细微，关于生命体最小单位——基因的各项研究也逐步走进了大众的视线。基因指的是具有编码功能的核苷酸序列，记录着生命体的所有信息，也是生命的传承载体。通过转录和翻译，完成了核苷酸序列到具有特定功能的蛋白质的表达，形成了各个组织器官，发挥着不同生理功能。在人类被解析的大约25 000个基因中，有超过3 000个基因突变与遗传病的发生有关，而更多与疾病相关的基因突变正在被迅速地发现。基因的有义突变，可能会引发遗传性疾病或细胞癌变，这些疾病无疑对人的生命造成了巨大威胁。随着病理遗传基础知识的提升，提高了我们对疾病机理的认识，也指导了治疗的方向。尽管人类在药物研发上投入了巨大的成本，但是至今只有少数的遗传疾病可通过小分子化合物来治愈。科研人员正探索着如何从基因层面克服遗传性疾病，目前也取得一定的进展和临床上的治疗。基因治疗（Gene therapy）是指通过基因置换、增补等方法将目的基因导入受体细胞，定向的替换或敲除致病基因，补偿缺陷基因功能或增强原基因功能，从而达到治疗的效果。现今，由于测序成本大幅度下降和人类基因组计划的完成，基因治疗尤其是个性化精准治疗成为人类健康研究的主要焦点，特别是临床医学和靶点治疗方面[1]。

基于核酸酶的基因编辑技术经历了三代变革，第一代是人工介导的锌指核酸酶技术（Zinc finger nucleases，ZFNs）[2-3]，第二代是类转录激活因子效应核酸酶技术（Transcription activator-like effectors nucleases，TALENs）[4-5]，第三代则是目前运用最广泛的成簇规律性间隔短回文重复序列及其相关蛋白技术（Clustered regularly interspaced short palindromic repeats – CRISPR-associated9，CRISPR-Cas9）[6-7]和基于CRISPR-Cas9单碱基编辑技术（Base editor，BE）[8-9]。ZFNs和TALENs基因编辑技术是利用设计的可识别特定DNA序列的效应蛋白与具有剪切功能的Fok I 核酸酶相融合，实现靶向位点的编辑。CRISPR-Cas9 系统是由识别靶向位点的单链引导RNA（sgRNA）与具有核酸内切酶功能的Cas9蛋白组成的复合体行使定点编辑。基于CRISPR-Cas9系统的BE技术则实现了单核酸的定向编辑。CRISPR-Cas9系统是由 sgRNA 特异性识别靶向位点，设计相对简单，高效精准，且成本低，因此，该技术在基础研究、医学探索和临床治疗中得到了广泛应用。基因编辑技术不仅在基因表达调控和功能研究，细胞动物模型的构建，癌基因靶向药物的设计筛选上展开利用，在基因治疗中也具有潜在的优势和发展前景，为艾滋病、肿瘤、单基因或多基因遗传病的治疗提供了更大的可能性。

1　基因传递系统的介绍

目前，应用和研究最为广泛的CRISPR-Cas9基因编辑技术支持质粒DNA、RNA和蛋白质这3种水平上的传递策略。传递编码Cas9蛋白和sgRNA的质粒DNA具有无须多次转染、方便快捷、稳定性高的优势（图1.1 Strategy Ⅰ）。相比而言，传递可以表达Cas9蛋白的mRNA和sgRNA（图1.1 Strategy Ⅱ）则有更低的脱靶率，而传递Cas9蛋白-sgRNA复合体（图1.1 Strategy Ⅲ）有较低的免疫原性，且不存在将CRISPR基因永久整合到宿主基因组的潜在问题[12]。随着近几年纳米技术的发展，CRISPR-Cas9系统的病毒和非病毒载体在体内和体外都有效地实现了向细胞和组织的递送，纳米载体逐渐成为CRISPR-Cas9系统基因治疗的潜在工具，新兴的递送策略也使得CRISPR-Cas9系统的递送更加成熟。

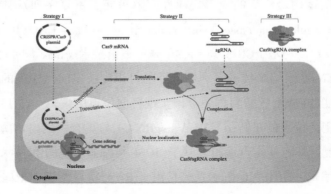

图 1.1　使用 CRISPR-Cas9 系统编辑基因的三种不同策略[12]

如图1.1所示，第一种是最直接的方法——使用基于质粒的CRISPR-Cas9系统，该系统编码来自同一载体的Cas9蛋白和sgRNA，从而避免了不同成分的多次转染。该载体将表达Cas9蛋白和sgRNA，它们将在细胞内部形成Cas9-sgRNA复合体，以编辑基因组序列。第二种策略是递送Cas9 mRNA和sgRNA的混合物。Cas9 mRNA将在细胞中翻译为Cas9蛋白，从而转化为Cas9-sgRNA复合物。第三种策略是将Cas9-sgRNA复合物直接递送到细胞中。

将目的基因导入细胞的方法可分为病毒传递、非病毒传递和物理传递方法[10-13]。病毒传递方法通过构建含目的基因的病毒载体，经病毒蛋白包装后感染宿主细胞，使目的基因进入宿主细胞内复制并表达，常用的病毒载体包括反转录病毒（retrovirus，RV）、慢病毒（lentivirus，LV）、腺病毒（adenovirus，AdV）、腺相关病毒（adeno-associated virus，AAV）等。该传递方法在临床上可同时用于体内和体外的基因编辑（图1.2）[13]。病毒介导的基因传递是目前最有效的基因传送方法，因为这些病毒载体可以提供组织趋向性，同时也可能引发插入诱变、免疫原性以及致癌作用等相关潜在问题。

非病毒传递则是不通过病毒作为转运载体，通过将目的基因注射至体内靶组织，使其进入靶向细胞复制表达。基于非病毒材料的递送载体具有比病毒载体低的毒性和免疫原性的潜力，但传递效率低是该传递方法的一大挑战。带负电荷的DNA和其他核酸可以与阳离子材料静电复合，形成纳米颗粒（nanoparticle），随后通过各种机制被细胞内吞，包括受体介导的内吞作用和吞噬作用[11]。用于核酸递送的最成功的阳离子材料类有天然存在的和合成的不同聚合物（如聚乙烯亚胺和环糊精）和不同的脂质类。目前，脂质纳米颗粒（lipid nanoparticles）和细胞内源物外泌体（exosome）作为非病毒传递方法被广泛应用在运送ZFNs、TALENs和CRISPR系统到不同的细胞和动物模型中[13]。虽然取得一定的研究进展和临床治疗效果，但它们的应用还面临很多问题，例如递送容量、药理问题等。

物理传递（不带载体的传递）则是利用物理方法将DNA序列或者蛋白质传递到靶向细胞或组织中，常用的方法有电穿孔（Electroporation）和流体动力注射（hydrodynamic injection）。在离体疗法中，电穿孔可在细胞膜上产生瞬时孔，从而使DNA和蛋白质进入细胞。对于体内治疗，利用流体动力注射未包装的DNA序列可以有效转染小鼠肝细胞，但出于安全性考虑，限制了在人体上应用该方法。另外，也可以利用物理方法将核酸直接注射到胚胎或合子中，但对人类胚胎基因组的编辑仍然存在很大争议。鉴于这些限制，用于基因编辑的可产生临床翻译的体内疗法仍需要病毒或非病毒递送载体。因此，该传递方法在此将不再详细讲解。

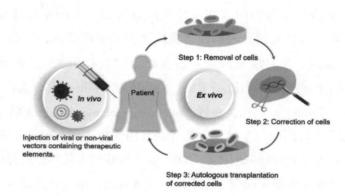

图 1.2　临床上体内和体外的基因编辑过程 [13]

如图1.2所示，右边是体外编辑疗法，目标细胞从患者体内分离、处理和编辑，再移植回患者体内。为了获得治疗成功，目标细胞必须能够在体外存活并在移植后返回目标组织。而左边是体内编辑疗法，工程化核酸酶通过病毒或非病毒方法传递，并直接注射到患者体内以产生全身或靶向组织的作用。

2　病毒载体

病毒载体顾名思义是利用病毒体积小、结构简单、感染快的优点进行分子感染，将带有遗传物质的目的基因转入靶向细胞。病毒载体运送目的基因以提供各种基于核酸治疗方法的研究已经有三十多年，其中一些已经被批准用于临床治疗[11, 14]。尽管存在着安全隐患和可能引入不可预料的突变的可能性，但病毒传递系统是迄今为止传递带有目的基因的质粒到靶向细胞和组织中最有效的系统[15-17]。因此，病毒载体已经被广泛地用于传递构建的CRISPR-Cas9质粒，应用于基础研究、基因疗法和疫苗设计，为这些领域提供了新的思路。在临床治疗上，对病毒的选择主要取决于转基因表达的效率、病毒产生的难易程度、安全性、毒性和稳定性。目前用作载体病毒的类型有：逆转录病毒、腺病毒及其相关病毒和慢病毒等。

2.1　逆转录病毒

逆转录病毒（retrovirus，RV）是一种单链RNA病毒，它能够在逆转录酶的作用下将RNA转变成cDNA，再在蛋白酶作用下进行DNA复制、转录、翻译等的一类病毒。逆转录病毒载体是根据逆转录病毒的特性设计出的一种病毒表达载体。逆转录病毒RNA基因组的核心部分包括三个编码蛋白质的基因：gag（编码病毒的核心蛋白）、pol（编码逆转录酶）和env（编码病毒的被膜糖蛋白），其结构基因的缺失不会影响其他部分的活性[18]。逆转录病毒具有强启动子，能够高效稳定表达外源基因，但它只能在分裂细胞内复制，因此只能感染分裂细胞。有的逆转录病毒还带有癌基因，有致癌性。因此，科研人员根据逆转录病毒的一些特性设计出了具有复制缺陷的病毒载体，使其能够特异性的携带特异目的基因的表达载体。

早期的逆转录病毒大多基于禽类病毒衍生而来，现在主要以一种肿瘤反转录病毒——Moloney小鼠白血病病毒构建而成[19]。它能感染多种不同种类生物的细胞，成功率非常高，甚至可以达到100%，有非常理想的临床效果。作为首例被用于临床基因治疗的病毒载体，逆转录病毒载体具有转染效率高，表达稳定持久的特点，但其容量较小，只能感染分裂细胞，且存在插入突变风险，不适用于治疗非致死性疾病。Mason[20]等使用逆转录病毒将*BMP-7*基因导入兔BMSCs，扩增培养后结合聚乙酸支架实现疾病的治疗，并取得了良好的效果。2017年，世界首批内源性逆转录病毒灭活猪诞生，从根本上解决了猪器官用于人体移植的异种病毒传播风险，将其逐渐发展成为最优质的基因治疗载体之一[21]。

在CRISPR-Cas9系统中，逆转录病毒开启了运用病毒载体进行临床治疗的大门，经过研究人员的不断深入的研究，不同病毒载体传递CRISPR-Cas9系统的作用体系被挖掘利用，使基因编辑技术攻克癌症和各种遗传性疾病逐渐成为可能。由于无法控制病毒载体在患者体内转录后是否产生毒性，且会随机整合，在人体临床试验中仍存在隐患，不能广泛的进行临床治疗。逆转录病毒载体的容量较小，只能整合7kb以下的外源基因。但逆转录病毒载体对建立治疗方案模型及后续研究方向提供了有意义的参考。

2.2　慢病毒

慢病毒（Lentivirus）是属于逆转录病毒科的RNA病毒，由于其感染人体的淋巴和巨噬细胞后，经过较长的潜伏期后才出现临床症状，因此被称为慢病毒[22]。利用慢病毒作为目的基因传递到靶向细胞的载体已经被广泛应用到基因治疗上。慢病毒载体最早是由1型人类免疫缺陷病毒（human immunodeficiency virus-1，HIV-1）改造而来的。除了具有温和的免疫原性和转导基因的长期表达外，慢病毒的最大优势是其高干扰效率，这一优势对肝脏、大脑和肌肉等组织中的基因编辑至关重要[23]。改造的慢病毒载体不含有多个和病毒活性有关的序列结构，进入人体细胞后不会引起免疫反应。在临床应用上构建慢病毒载体通常需要两种不同类型的质粒，一种是包装质粒，可以编码产生病毒颗粒所需的结构蛋白和酶，另一种质粒则包含外源遗传物质用于基因编辑，如Cas9编码序列和sgRNA[24]。

慢病毒区别于一般的逆转录病毒载体，可以感染分裂细胞和非分裂细胞，并具有较高的重组效率和稳定性，其介导的基因治疗已经在临床研究中取得了可喜的成果。2002年慢病毒载体首次被批准用于临床试验，首次获批的临床试验是抗HIV病毒的RNA治疗，实验证明通过慢病毒载体进行治疗具有短期疗效，并已进入临床Ⅰ期试验[25]。慢病毒载体携带的目的基因在大多数Wiskott-Aldrich综合征患者的造血干细胞中体现出稳定的、较高水平的重组率，以及在肾上腺皮质营养不良患者体内体现出90%以上的重组率[26-27]。另外，中国贵州医科大学的Zhang Fei等研究人员，使用慢病毒转染兔骨髓间充质干细胞（bone marrow mesenchymal stem cells，BMSCs）过表达成纤维细胞生长因子（fibroblast growth factor，FGF-2）基因联合异种抗原提取的松质骨（xenogeneic antigen-extracted cancellous bone，XACB）来构建组织工程骨，用于治疗缺血性股骨头坏死，有效地促进了血管再生和提高了修复效果[28]。另外，慢病毒载体也已被广泛应用于神经退行性疾病、帕金森病、镰状细胞性贫血、地中海贫血、HIV等疾病的治疗试验[29-33]。利用慢病毒介导的CRISPR-Cas9传递系统在体内和体外均取得了成功的应用。

虽然慢病毒的研究已经取得了很大的进展，但有报道指出用慢病毒载体进行基因编辑时会使病毒DNA整合到宿主基因组上，并由此导致非靶基因的突变，因此，慢病毒在临床上的应用存在一定的安全隐患[34]。在常规的基因治疗中，慢病毒的整合酶依赖机制可以使目的基因稳定表达，保持细胞遗传缺陷的互补性。但当慢病毒载体运输CRISPR-Cas9系统时，Cas9和sgRNA的持续存在可能导致较高的脱靶效应，使慢病毒的整合能力下降。另一问题是慢病毒的滴度不够高，根据已有的报道显示大多数实验室包装的慢病毒滴度均在 108IU/mL左右，较难满足临床需求[35]。因此，利用慢病毒作为运输载体在基因编辑的过程中利弊共存，它在靶向细胞运输基因编辑元件时有较高的稳定性和可靠性，同时，它在安全性和脱靶效应等方面也存在着一定的隐患。

2.3 腺病毒

腺病毒（adenovirus，AdV）是于1953年从人类的腺样体组织中首次被分离出来的，是引起呼吸道感染的常见原因[36]。目前有超过89种公认的人类腺病毒基因型，基于其基因特点的不同可以归为7类，命名为人腺病毒A至G（HAdVA至HAdVG），新的腺病毒类型还在不断涌现[37-39]。腺病毒的直径为 70～100nm，是一种无包膜的具有二十面体蛋白质外壳的双链DNA病毒，长度在26～45kb之间，其序列两端均形成一个发夹结构，称为反向末端重复序列（inverted terminal repeats，ITR）[37, 40, 42]。腺病毒作为载体传递目的基因具有许多优势：（Ⅰ）这些病毒易操作和生成；（Ⅱ）可以维持稳定的高滴度原种以重复利用；（Ⅲ）它们可以感染分裂和非分裂细胞；（Ⅳ）它们能以高感染性感染广泛的宿主。外源基因作为附加体被腺病毒载体表达，在体内具有较低的基因毒性[41]。腺病毒载体最高可插入8kb的外源片段，具有较高的转染效率和表达水平，但由于其高滴度会在宿主体内中引起显著的免疫反应[42]。腺病毒的表达不需要整合到宿主细胞基因组中，仅能瞬间表达，因此，当腺病毒载体应用到临床试验时，无法实现长期的治疗。

腺病毒载体在临床试验上已经被广泛地应用，全球已经获批了2 000多项基于腺病毒载体的基因疗法临床试验[42-44]。1992年，美国国家癌症研究所（National Cancer Institute）的Jaffe H. A.等研究人员首次成功地实现了使用腺病毒载体进行体内基因治疗，研究表明腺病毒载体能在肝细胞内传递和表达目的基因，也证实了该载体可用于肝脏疾病的基因治疗[45]。腺病毒载体在基因治疗方面应用最多的应该是癌症的治疗[41, 43, 46-47]。已有研究表明通过腺病毒可成功将肿瘤抑制基因p53和p16递送到肿瘤细胞中，而首次获批的腺病毒基因治疗就是利用腺病毒递送p53基因来抑制肿瘤生长[48]。自杀基因疗法和前体药物疗法也可以作为治疗肿瘤的方法，其中，自杀治疗是利用腺病毒将无毒的药物递送到靶细胞中并代谢成有毒药物，使细胞死亡。除此之外，腺病毒载体也被广泛应用于干细胞分化、艾滋病、心血管疾病和肺结核等疾病的研究中[49-52]。

2.4　腺相关病毒

腺相关病毒（adeno-associated virus，AAV）是由美国匹茨堡大学（University of Pittsburgh）的Robert W. Atchison等研究人员于1965年首次从猿猴腺病毒制剂中分离出来的含有DNA的小颗粒[53]。他们研究发现腺相关病毒在抗原上不同于腺病毒，而且只有跟腺病毒同时接种时才能在细胞培养物中复制，因此是一种缺陷型病毒。腺相关病毒是一种无包膜的具有二十面体蛋白质外壳的、DNA基因组长度约为4.7kb的单链DNA病毒，直径约为22nm，是一种非常微小的病毒[54]。由于其具有非致病性、低免疫原性、广泛的血清型特异性，以及感染分裂和非分裂细胞的能力，因此，腺相关病毒是目前应用最广泛的病毒载体[55-56]。目前，已经有200多种不同的分子工程设计的和天然存在的腺相关病毒变体[57-58]。2012年，欧洲批准了首个基于腺相关病毒的基因治疗药物Glybera用于脂蛋白脂肪酶缺乏症患者，这表明了该病毒在基因治疗方面有着广阔的应用前景，同时也在转运基于质粒的CRISPR-Cas9系统上有了广泛的应用[59-60]。

编码化脓链球菌Cas9（SpCas9）蛋白和sgRNA的序列约为4.2kb，腺相关病毒载体整合外源片段的长度限制在4.5 kb以内，因此用腺相关病毒转运CRSIPR-Cas9的最大限制是其承载量不足。一种解决方案是使用截短的SpCas9或金黄色葡萄球菌Cas9（SaCas9），SaCas9的基因编辑效率与SpCas9相似，但尺寸较小，而使用截短的SpCas9的缺陷是其活性较低[61]。美国麻省理工学院和哈佛大学广泛研究所（Broad Institute of MIT and Harvard）的张锋实验室研究人员将编码SaCas9蛋白和gRNA的序列包装到AAV中，靶向小鼠的PCSK9，实现了约40%的基因编辑效率，而且伴随着PCSK9和血清中总胆固醇水平的显著下降，并没有表现出明显的毒性[62]。另一项研究中，科学家们将SaCas9和多种sgRNA整合到腺相关病毒，并转运到靶向位点，显示出约60%的基因编辑效率[63]。

另一种解决方案是使用双腺相关病毒载体分别传递编码Cas9的DNA和sgRNA，以克服单个腺相关病毒载体的整合片段长度的限制。张锋实验室的Lukasz Swiech等使用两种分离的腺相关病毒载体分别传递SpCas9和sgRNA到靶向小鼠大脑细胞，成功的改变了靶向单个基因和多个基因[64]。这个双载体系统也用作转运CRISPR-Cas9来治疗小鼠模型中的代谢性肝病[65]。研究人员用一个载体转运SaCas9基因，另一个载体转运sgRNA和供体模版基因，用这个双载体系统纠正了小鼠肝细胞中10%的突变。尽管这种双载体策略得到了成功，但将两个腺相关病毒载体注入同一个靶向细胞仍具有挑战性。

第三种解决方案是由张锋实验室的Bernd Zetche等人提出的，它们设计了一种AAV介导的split-Cas9系统，该系统可以在西罗莫司（rapamycin）的作用下自发地在细胞内部自动组装Cas9蛋白。他们鉴定出11个Cas9蛋白中的潜在分裂位点，可以将Cas9蛋白分为C端和N端两部分，西罗莫司诱导这两部分片段重组为全长Cas9蛋白，随后可编辑HEK293FT细胞中的基因[66]。腺病毒载体的递送系统已在临床治疗上得以应用，但CRISPR-Cas9系统的体内编辑效率明显低于体外编辑，所以有效的基因编辑仍然是一个很大的挑战。

在不同的动物研究中，腺相关病毒已经被用于治疗囊性纤维化[67]、皮肤烧伤和血友病[68-71]等疾病，研究人员还发现该病毒能在不同的组织和细胞中稳定表达，包括脑、心脏、肝脏、肌肉和视网膜细胞等。腺相关病毒能广泛地感染各种不同的组织，很大程度上是因为其不同的血清型的衣壳具有差异性，能够感染不同的细胞组织。例如，最常用的AAV2对硫酸乙酰肝素蛋白聚糖（Heparan sulfate proteoglycan，HSPG）受体具有较高的亲和力，而这种受体存在于多种类型的细胞中，因此AAV2应用最广泛[72]。AAV5通常与血小板源生长因子受体结合，这类受体常见于脑、肺和视网膜细胞中，因此，AAV5更倾向于治疗脑、肺及眼睛相关的疾病[73]。

这四类病毒载体是病毒类载体运送CRISPR-Cas9系统的"主力军"，也有应用在临床试验或治疗上，其他未开发的病毒仍然具有被探索成为载体的潜力，例如不同类型的疱疹病毒，在控制其致病性后可以成为另外的载体病毒，为其他病症的治疗带来思路。

3　非病毒载体

　　非病毒传递方法具有整合和转移较大目的序列的潜力。尽管目前已发现并开发了各种合成载体，但在临床研究阶段仅使用了一小部分非病毒载体。而相对于病毒载体，非病毒载体具有瞬时表达模式，以及可重复应用和可提高传递效率的独特优势。在过去的几十年中，纳米药物已成功地引入临床试验，并且药物研究的不断发展正在创造出更复杂的药物。各种各样的非病毒纳米粒子，如脂质体，聚合物纳米粒子和无机纳米粒子等已经显示出在体内和体外传递基因和蛋白质药物的高效性[74-75]。肿瘤组织通常发展为血管渗漏和不良的淋巴引流，从而使纳米颗粒通过渗漏的血管扩散和积累到肿瘤组织中[76]。另外，将基因或蛋白质配制成纳米颗粒可保护其在生物环境中不被降解，增强细胞吸收不渗透细胞的治疗剂，并延长静脉内给药后的代谢循环[77-78]。因此，非病毒纳米颗粒为传递基因编辑系统提供了有效的平台。

3.1　纳米药物（nanomedicines）的介绍

　　20世纪60年代科学家首次提出脂质体的概念，经过30多年的研究，第一个脂质体纳米药物阿霉素Doxil是一种针对HIV肿瘤的治疗药物[79]，并于1995年由美国FDA批准上市。随着科技的不断创新，纳米技术蓬勃发展，纳米药物也迅速发展起来。常用的纳米药物技术方法是将药物分布在各种纳米载体中，例如固体脂质、多聚体纳米粒等，它可以控制降解的时间、提供生物利用度、减少对正常组织的细胞毒性，从而为基因治疗提供可行性。由于其可行性和多样性，为纳米技术和药物传递的研发提供了广阔的空间。

纳米药物将纳米材料和药物结合起来，在保证传统药物药效的情况下充分利用了纳米材料具有的优势[76]。纳米材料本身的多样性，使研究者可以根据需求进行纳米药物的研发或改进。纳米药物对肿瘤、炎症等具有特异的靶向性，因此被主要用于肿瘤、免疫性疾病的药物开发。为了解决靶向效率低等问题，研究者利用环境特异性来提高运输效率，通过控制药物粒径和表面电荷来增强载体扩散能力，或是将较为成熟的分子靶向和载体靶向相结合构成逐级靶向[81]。关于纳米药物的生物安全和毒理学的研究也取得了突破性的进展，如碳纳米管等明星材料的安全性研究已经取得了重大进步[82]。随着科研人员的研究发展，将来会有更加智能化和更多类型的纳米载体和新纳米药物出现，以弥补目前药物研究的短板。

3.2　脂质纳米颗粒载体（Lipid nanoparticles，LNs）

脂质体是合成的球形囊泡，最小的脂质体大约30nm，最大的可以达到几微米，脂质体的大小和表面成分会影响巨噬细胞对它的有效摄取量和靶向递送到血管壁的能力。在基于脂质体的系统中，脂质纳米颗粒在体外和体内均可以作为基因和RNA干扰系统的载体[83-86]。与其他非病毒载体相比，脂质纳米颗粒表现出若干优势，例如低或无体内毒性、长期稳定性好等，这与耐受性良好的生理脂质组成有关，通常被批准用于人体药物制剂中，通过经济且无溶剂的技术进行生产，或者可以进行高压灭菌或消毒的方法[87-88]。脂质纳米颗粒代表了最常用的核酸转运系统之一。带负电荷的核酸通过静电相互作用与带正电荷的脂质复合，形成脂质纳米颗粒，从而保护核酸免受核酸酶侵害，并通过内吞作用或巨胞饮作用进入靶细胞。

脂质纳米颗粒已被研究用于将CRISPR-Cas9系统递送至不同细胞[7, 89]，用于治疗疾病或建立基因敲除的动物模型[90-91]。当用于递送CRISPR-Cas9系统时，有两种主要的脂质纳米颗粒使用方法：传递Cas9和sgRNA遗传物质（质粒DNA或mRNA），或传递Cas9-sgRNA核糖核蛋白复合物（ribonucleoprotein complexes，RNP）。如果递送Cas9蛋白的mRNA和sgRNA，则该方法在功能上类似于显微注射[92]。同时，有几个研究小组在用脂质纳米颗粒传递Cas9-sgRNA核糖核蛋白复合物上取得了成功[93-94]。CRISPR-Cas9系统比较适合复合体的递送，因为Cas9-sgRNA作为核糖核蛋白复合物具有高度阴离子性，这使得它们可以利用递送核酸的方法进行包装。

通过脂质纳米颗粒递送CRISPR-Cas9系统也存在很多限制。首先，需要考虑传递时细胞内部和外部的障碍。纳米颗粒通过细胞表面后，通常被包裹在内体中。被包裹的内容物可以非常快速地被细胞引导进入溶酶体途径，导致内容物被降解。因此，传递物必须能够逸出内含体。同样的，如果Cas9-sgRNA复合体能够逃脱内含体，也必须要转移到细胞核才能实现基因编辑，这也可能是潜在的失败点。通过脂质纳米颗粒递送CRISPR-Cas9系统的传递率较低。然而，美国塔夫茨大学（Tufts University）的Ming Wang等研究人员利用纸质纳米颗粒在传送CRISPR-sgRNA核糖核蛋白复合体后，在体外细胞中达到70%的修饰效率，他们用的是经过严格筛选确定的最优化的脂质构建的脂质体系统实现的[94]。美国哈佛大学的John A. Zuris等研究人员将带有负电荷的绿色荧光蛋白（green florescence protein，GFP）与Cas9蛋白融合，脂质纳米颗粒递送由修饰的Cas9蛋白和sgRNA制成的核糖核蛋白复合体，经过一种处理后，可在培养的人类细胞中诱导高达80%的基因编辑。同时，他们实验证明，修饰的Cas9-sgRNA核糖核蛋白复合体在小鼠体内可以递送到小鼠的内耳，并在毛细胞中编辑20%的目的基因[93]。脂质纳米颗粒就像病毒颗粒一样，会因为传递的性质和大小以及目标细胞类型而影响转染效率[10]。而与基于质粒的CRISPR-Cas9相比，传递CRISPR-sgRNA核糖核蛋白复合体通常显示出更高的基因编辑效率和更少的脱靶效应。因此，已经投入相当大的努力来开发用于核糖核蛋白复合体的新脂质纳米颗粒[12]。

目前，最常用的脂质纳米颗粒是可商购的Lipofectamine，这是一种阳离子脂质体制剂，可与带负电荷的核酸复合，从而使复合物与带负电荷的细胞膜融合并发生内吞作用。Lipofectamine已用于将编码Cas9和sgRNA的质粒DNA递送至人类多能干细胞，例如构建了免疫缺陷，着丝粒区域不稳定性和面部异常综合征（Facial anomalies syndrome，ICF）的模型，转染效率为63%，用具有7个sgRNA和Cas9核酸酶的多复合体转染人细胞，还用于纠正培养的囊性纤维化患者肠干细胞中的囊性纤维化跨膜导体受体基因座等[95-97]。

提高非病毒载体的递送效率是在运送基因编辑技术上需要解决的一个问题。美国得克萨斯大学西南医学中心（University of Texas Southwestern Medical Center）的Jason B. Miller等研究人员设计了一类两性离子氨基脂质（zwitterionic amino lipids，ZALs）和一个独特的共传递Cas9 mRNA 和sgRNA的长RNA。ZAL纳米颗粒（ZAL nanoparticle，ZNP）可以递送低剂量（15 nM）长sgRNA，使细胞蛋白表达量降低了90%以上[97]。为促进载体逃脱内含体，提高基因编辑效率，中国科学院（The Chinese Academy of Sciences）的Liu Ji等设计、筛选出一种集成有二硫键的脂质纳米颗粒BAMEA-O16B（含有3个二硫键），可以有效地将Cas9 mRNA和sgRNA递送到细胞中，同时于还原性细胞内环境释放RNA，以便在mRNA递送后24h内进行基因组编辑。结果表明，使用BAMEA-O16B同时递送Cas9 mRNA和sgRNA可以使人类胚胎肾细胞的绿色荧光蛋白（GFP）表达效率高达90%。静脉注射该脂质纳米颗粒可以将小鼠血清PCSK9水平调低至对照组的20%[98]。

类脂化合物在体内无法降解，会带来严重的不良反应，设计可降解的脂质或类脂化合物可以进一步提高载体安全性。美国俄亥俄州立大学（Ohio State University）的Xinfu Zhang等设计和合成了一系列具有酯基的可生物降解脂质样化合物，用于传递编码mRNA的Cas9。他们合成的两个先导材料，线性酯链结构的N-甲基-1，3丙二胺（N-methyl-1，3-propanediamine，MPA）-A和具有分支酯链结构的MPA-Ab，显示出可调节的生物降解速率。同时，证明了MPA-A和MPA-Ab在体外和体内有效传递Cas9 mRNA[99]。因此，这些可生物降解的类脂质纳米材料作为生物和治疗应用的基因组编辑传递工具，值得进一步的研究和发展。美国Intellia Therapeutics公司的Jonathan D.Finn等研究人员合成了一种可电离脂质LP01，具有较好的生物可降解性和相容性。LNP-INT01（LP01制备的脂质纳米颗粒）单次给药后即可对小鼠肝细胞中甲状腺素

（transthyretin，Ttr）基因进行编辑，使血清蛋白水平降低97%以上，而且作用效果持续了12个月以上[100]。这些结果是通过可生物降解且耐受性良好的脂质纳米颗粒递送系统获得的，该递送系统与具有化学修饰模式的sgRNA结合，这对高水平的体内活性至关重要。

脂质体是抗肿瘤纳米药物的主要剂型之一，也是临床转化最成功的一类纳米药物。脂质体是第一个被FDA授予IND资格并在临床试验中进行研究的纳米药物[101]。纳米递药系统能同时荷载多个药物，并可以改变原有药动学特征，确保所载的多个药物从给药开始到进入肿瘤细胞都能维持合适的比例，有利于药物间协同作用的发挥。Vyxeos是美国FDA于2017年批准的第一个含有阿糖胞苷（Cytarabine）和道诺霉素（Daunorubicin）两种原料药的脂质体产品。在针对骨髓性白血病的Ⅲ期临床研究中，比较了脂质体产品与标准阿糖胞苷–道诺霉素（5：1）方案。与对照组（游离阿糖胞苷和道诺霉素）相比，Vyxeos提高了整体存活率，并表现出类似的安全性[102]。2015年到2018年期间，国内也有5家药企的脂质体注射液成功上市，分别是南京绿叶制药的注射用紫杉醇脂质体，上海上药新亚药业的注射用两性霉素B脂质体，石药集团、常州金远和上海复旦张江的盐酸多柔比星脂质体注射液[103-104]。目前的脂质体产品设计和工艺可能还需要进一步的改进。然而，对于治疗用脂质体的生物相容性、生物降解性和毒性安全性的认识也促进了未来脂质体产品的开发[105]。

4 外泌体及其在医学研究上的开发和应用

4.1 外泌体的介绍

1983年，加拿大麦吉尔大学（McGill University）的Rose M. Johnstone等研究人员在研究成熟过程中的网织红细胞中首次发现了分泌到细胞外的膜性囊泡，并于1987年通过超速离心的方法分离到该囊泡，命名为外泌体（exosome）[106]。外泌体是由活细胞吞噬异源物质后以出芽方式向内凹陷形成含有多个小泡的多泡体（vesicular body，vB），与细胞膜融合后释放到细胞外的小囊泡，直径为30～100nm，是细胞间信号传导的载体[107]。外泌体通过细胞外刺激，微生物攻击或其他应激条件的诱导，可由间充质干细胞、肿瘤细胞、免疫细胞、人羊膜上皮细胞、内皮祖细胞等人体中不同类型的细胞释放，广泛分布于各种体液中，如唾液、腹水、心包积液、尿液、羊水、乳汁、脑脊液和血液等，参与细胞凋亡、细胞通讯、炎症反应、血管新生和肿瘤生长等过程[108]。

外泌体以往曾被认为是细胞分泌的垃圾。外泌体中携带脂质、蛋白质和遗传物质，其中蛋白质和遗传物质是其发挥生物学功能的有效成分。外泌体的膜与细胞一样，是磷脂双分子层，其形成机制非常简单，简而言之，即是"内吞-融合-外排"（图4.1）[108]。从1983年首次发现外泌体至今，已有30多年的历史，最初被认为是细胞分泌的"垃圾"，是细胞排泄废物的一种方式。但随着研究的深入，科学家们发现细胞囊泡运输的调节机制，在细胞间通讯和细胞免疫应答中发挥重要作用。2013年的诺贝尔生理学或医学奖授予给美国科学家詹姆斯·罗斯曼（James Rothman）、兰迪·谢克曼（Randy Schekman）和德国科学家托马斯·苏德霍夫（Thomas C.Südhof），以表彰他们在发现细胞囊泡运输系统及其运行调节机制研究中做出的杰出贡献。有趣的是，罗斯曼和谢克曼博士早在2002年就因相同成果获得被称为诺贝尔奖先导的拉斯克（Lasker）奖，许多科学家认为他们的诺奖"迟到"了。更有学者认为，过去一二十年间的高通量测序和基因表达谱检测的热潮一度改变了整个生物学的研究进程，削弱了对包括细胞内囊泡转运系统在内的基本细胞生物学应有的重视。本次诺奖的颁布在很大程度上，使人们回归到对细胞基本生理过程的关注。但不可否认，正是以核酸测序为代表的高通量组学分析技术的日趋成熟，使得对细胞囊泡的研究进入了空前的繁荣阶段，并将深刻影响人类疾病的研究，开启了外泌体研究的新时代[109-110]。

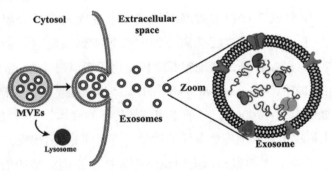

图 4.1　外泌体生物发生的示意图

如图4.1所示，首先形成了包含外泌体的多囊泡内体（MVE）。 MVE可以与质膜融合，将外泌体释放到细胞外基质中，也可以与溶酶体融合降解。外泌体包含蛋白质、DNA、RNA和表面膜蛋白，这些蛋白对供体细胞具有特异性，而不仅限于细胞表面蛋白。

外泌体和微囊泡、凋亡小体明显不同，有鲜明的特点和潜在价值，时至今日，已逐步成为科研热点。这种机体内普遍存在的纳米级被膜结构能够参与细胞间的物质交换和信息交流，在多种生理和病理过程中发挥重要作用。在外周血、尿液、唾液、腹水、羊水等体液中具有很高的丰度，而不同组织来源的外泌体在组成和功能方面存在差异，同时这种差异受到细胞外基质和微环境的动态调控。肿瘤来源或肿瘤相关的外泌体是调控肿瘤发生发展的重要途径之一，这使得外泌体在生理和病理过程中都发挥重要的作用。

外泌体作为一种内源性胞外囊泡，包含了复杂的RNA和蛋白质，可作为新一代天然纳米级药物递送系统。外泌体中的脂类分子主要是细胞质膜及其类似成分，另有一些与来源细胞相关的特殊脂类。这些脂类分子不仅参与维持外泌体的形态，还可以作为信号分子参与许多生物学过程，如对Notch等一些关键肿瘤生存信号通路的抑制，引起细胞凋亡，以及对前列腺素、磷酸激酶A2、C和D等一些中间信号分子的传递，参与细胞间通讯。基于外泌体的药物载体系统，可解决传统纳米药物载体难以同时兼顾药物传递效率与生物相容性、潜在毒性和免疫反应等难题。然而，基于外泌体的药物载体，仍需要克服半衰期短、缺乏特异性靶向能力和细胞内传递效率低等困难[110]。因此，通过表面改造或用功能配体修饰来改善外泌体的输送性能具有显著意义，是促进外泌体临床应用的必要条件。目前外泌体的改造策略主要有"细胞工程"和"外泌体工程"两种。外泌体由供体细胞分泌，因此可通过"细胞工程"改变供体细胞遗传特性，传递到细胞膜的分子自然地整合在出芽的囊泡中，而内化到细胞内部的物质可以被包装到分泌的外泌体。"外泌体工程"则是直接操纵外泌体来实现表面功能化。

"细胞工程"改造外泌体是在细胞层面进行的研究，通过生物合成过程，借助供体细胞自身产生蛋白质的机制来改造外泌体，成为实验可应用的特殊外泌体。根据其来源的细胞类型和分化状态，作为一种新的和更复杂的细胞间通讯形式，外泌体在不同的生理和病理过程中发挥作用。外泌体还携带多种分子成分参与细胞通讯、细胞迁移、血管新生和肿瘤细胞生长等生理和病理过程。据报道，外泌体分泌的微小RNA（miRNA）可在现阶段帮助诊断早期癌症，尤其在肺癌、结肠直肠癌、前列腺癌等癌症诊断中可作为诊断及预后的生物标志物[110]。目前可以通过修饰和改造对外泌体进行加工，修饰方法可将细胞的膜蛋白、糖基以及脂质体进行修饰，分泌得到修饰后的外泌体；改造是基于脂质体，采用机械挤压、包装外源物质等方法，通过改造细胞后，分泌得到改造后的外泌体。"外泌体工程"是对外泌体表面改造或修饰功能配体，增强外泌体的药物载体系统的方法。外泌体配体的功能化可以减缓外泌体的清除和跨膜效率[111-112]。外泌体参与细胞通信等过程，具有毒性低、免疫原性低、生物相容性高、可穿过血脑屏障等特点，可作为药物载体发挥治疗作用。

4.2　外泌体转载药物的方式

药物纳米载体的研究已经取得了一定成绩[113]，另外，随着合成化学技术的发展，也使基于药物递送的治疗性纳米颗粒呈现蓬勃发展的趋势，研究或应用较多的外源性载体包括有脂质体、纳米粒、微球等纳米颗粒新兴给药系统。目前已在药物的溶解性、化学和生物功能的稳定性和效能等方面做出改善，但这些纳米载体仍存在一些问题，例如针对病变组织，细胞靶向能力有限；纳米载体及其降解产物存在细胞毒性；能被单核吞噬系统的快速清除等，因此仅有少量被批准用于临床。为解决常规递送系统的局限性，越来越多的研究聚焦于开发更安全有效的内源性细胞或亚细胞结构的载体上。外源性载体在体外的物理化学性质稳定，但进入体内后，在血液循环中很快被网状内皮系统（reticuloendothelial system，RES）识别和清除，而且由于调理素、抗体等作用，有些载体易发生破裂，运载的药物会发生渗漏，从而影响稳定性及其在特定病灶部位的累积，极大地降低了外源性载体的有效性。

与这些合成载体相反，因为外泌体具有脂质双层结构，可通过电穿孔、共孵育、超声处理、超滤离心处理及挤出和冻融循环等技术将药物载入外泌体中，也可通过转染技术将miRNA递送进特定的细胞，使其分泌含微小RNA的外泌体。外泌体膜表面有各种蛋白分子，具有更好的生物相容性，能有效地针对病变组织、细胞，因此外泌体载体有希望克服人工合成载体带来的一系列问题。外泌体可通过细胞间信号转导接触远端受体细胞，也可通过定位于靶组织的能力选择性进入靶细胞，如胶质母细胞瘤分泌的外泌体膜表面含有小窝蛋白-1（caveolin-1），其通过抑制细胞外调节蛋白激酶1/2（extracellular regulated protein kinases1/2，ERK1/2）的激活负调控外泌体的内化。作为内源性载体，与外源性纳米载体相比，外泌体具有更低的免疫原性，可避免RES的吞噬，更有效地穿过许多药物难以穿透的血脑屏障。目前，外泌体载体的研究进展还处于实验室和临床试验阶段。不同组织细胞分泌的外泌体携带不同的生物学组分，赋予外泌体独特的生物学作用。基于其内源性、生物相容性和多功能特性，外泌体有望成为药物递送系统、免疫治疗和精准治疗的新手段，为相关的研究发展提供新思路。将外泌体最终应用于治疗，还要面对的挑战是如何有效地将药物加载入外泌体中。脂质体和其他合成载体可在合成过程中装载目标药物，而外泌体是从亲代细胞中产生的，因此它们必须在形成后立即装载药物或通过改造亲代细胞使其分泌目标药物。目前，这些方法导致外泌体中药物装载效率和稳定性不同。

4.2.1　药物与外泌体共孵育

自Sun等通过证明姜黄素孵育的方式实现了外泌体的被动加载，将外泌体与姜黄素共同孵育5min后，检测出每1g外泌体的负载量为29g姜黄素，并允许其在体内延迟释放，通过激活髓样细胞为受体细胞，干预免疫紊乱[114]。孵育加载药物存在效率不高的弊端，可能与外泌体本身已携带大量的蛋白质和核酸有关。目前，药物与外泌体进行孵育作为简单有效的负载方法被大家认同。Agrawal等探讨了乳源性的外泌体经口服递送紫杉醇（paclitaxel，PTX）代替静脉注射改善药物毒性的可能性。研究结果表明，负载PTX外泌体（Exo-PTC）经口服作用与人肺癌的荷瘤小鼠与同等剂量静脉注射PTX抑制作用无统计学差异，且经口服Exo-PTC全身毒性和免疫原性均较低[115]。

4.2.2　物理方式——电穿孔

装载药物到外泌体的物理方式——电穿孔是利用施加外部电场而形成亲水孔的过程，通过形成临时通道可将药物加载到外泌体中，外泌体膜完整性很快会恢复。电穿孔的参数易于控制，可将各种货物载入到外泌体中。由于外泌体中天然携带各种RNA，因此最常用的是将小分子干扰RNA（small interfering RNA，siRNA）整合到外泌体中。英国牛津大学（University of Oxford）的Lydia Alvarez-Erviti 等研究人员通过电穿孔将siRNA加载到树突状细胞（dendritic cell，DC）分泌的外泌体中，并成功运输siRNA至大脑中[116]。美国华盛顿大学（Washington University）的Joshua L. Hood等研究表明电穿孔加载RNA效率优于被动装载[117]。美国马里兰大学（University of Maryland）的Tek N. Lamichhane等证明了外泌体可通过电穿孔加载DNA并传递至受体细胞的能力，且线性、长度小于100p的DNA与外泌体结合效率更高，同时外泌体本身的大小也影响DNA装载效率[118]。迄今为止，RNA已被成功加载到外泌体中，且被证明可广泛应用，然而外泌体负载DNA潜在用途的研究相对较少。也有研究人员表明电穿孔会导致siRNA聚集，使得通过电穿孔加载药物到外泌体效率可能被高估[119]。

4.2.3　外泌体的转染

目前，已有市售的转染试剂可以有效地将siRNA加载到外泌体并成功传递至受体细胞。俄罗斯SFBI圣彼得堡核物理研究所（SFBI Petersburg Nuclear Physics Institute）在Tatyana A Shtam等研究人员通过共聚焦显微镜和流式细胞术证明了外泌体可以在体外将荧光标记的siRNA传递至受体细胞。他们将两种针对RAD51、RAD52的不同siRNA与脂质体转染试剂一起转入到外泌体中，并递送至靶细胞，证实了载有RAD51 siRNA的外泌体成功使癌细胞中RAD51基因沉默，引起受体癌细胞的大量生殖细胞死亡[120]。美国路易斯维尔大学（University of Louisville）的Anastasia Familtseva等为了将siRNA转染到外泌体中并成功递送至受体细胞的过程可视化，使用转染试剂将带有红色荧光标记的siRNA转染到小鼠主动脉内皮细胞（mouse aortic endothelial cell，MAEC）产生的外泌体中。与MAEC细胞孵育后发现荧光标记的siRNA成功递送至MAEC中，证实了基于转染试剂的有效性[121]。但该研究表明与电穿孔相比，使用转染剂的装载效率低，也无法从剩余的试剂中鉴定出负载siRNA的外泌体。考虑到化学转染的潜在毒性，基于转染的方法可能不适用于临床治疗。

4.2.4 "细胞工程"活化供体细胞

通过"细胞工程"改造供体细胞，使供体细胞活化，产生含有特定组成的外泌体也可以用作药物治疗。虽然这不是临床应用中最合适的选择，却也反映了外泌体生理中独特的现象。中国中山大学附属中山纪念医院的Lv Lihong等研究人员将HepG2细胞与不同抗癌药物（依托泊苷、卡铂、伊立替康、PTX）解育后，从HepG2细胞中释放的外泌体对人胰腺癌细胞系CFPAC-1表现出强大的抗增殖活性，并诱导了基于热休克蛋白免疫原性和特异性的NK细胞杀伤效应[122]。另一项研究表明，将姜黄素与RAW 264.7细胞共同孵育产生的外泌体在通过血脑屏障后激活蛋白激酶B糖原合成酶激酶3（protein kinase B/glycogen synthase kinase 3β，AKT/IGSK 3β）通路，抑制Tau蛋白磷酸化，防止神经元死亡，从而缓解阿尔兹海默病的症状[124]。

4.2.5 转染供体细胞

到目前为止，将治疗性药物装载到外泌体中应用最广泛的方法是转染产生外泌体的供体细胞。转染后的供体细胞可过表达特定基因，将其包裹在外泌体内或外泌体膜上，通过外泌体运输到靶向细胞[124]。中国中山大学附属中山纪念医院的Wen Zhuzhi等研究人员探索在缺氧条件下，由骨髓间充质干细胞（mesenchymal stem cell，MSC）衍生的外泌体中包含有miRNA，通过将miRNA传递至靶向同源性磷酸酶张力蛋白，磷酸化蛋白激酶B（phosphate and tesion homology deleted on chromosome ten/phosphorylated protein kinase B，PTEN/AKT）通路的细胞可抑制心肌细胞凋亡损伤[125]。中国天津医科大学的Zhang Haiyang等模拟肿瘤微环境，通过外泌体传递的miR-29a/c可以显著抑制胃癌细胞中的血管内皮生长因子（Vascular Endothelial Growth Factor，VEGF）的表达，从而抑制血管细胞的生长、转移和管形成[126]。他们的研究结果提供了通过使用含miRNA的外泌体阻断血管生成来控制肿瘤细胞生长的新型抗癌策略。然而，转染供体细胞会存在一定的细胞毒作用、特异性差和包装效率低等限制，需要进一步了解其潜在的毒性和攻克其缺陷，才能将该技术利用于临床试验中。

4.2.6　外泌体转载靶蛋白

外泌体转载药物的形式有多种，但低效率、复杂的纯化技术和潜在的毒性为临床试验应用带来了限制。2016年，韩国科学技术研究院（National Research University）的Nambin Yim等研究人员描述了一种新的用于靶蛋白在细胞内递送的工具，称为"通过光学可逆的蛋白-蛋白相互作用来加载蛋白的外泌体"（exosomes for protein loading via optically reversible protein - protein interactions，EXPLORs）。通过将受蓝光控制的可逆蛋白质-蛋白质相互作用模块与外泌体生物发生的内生过程整合，我们能够成功地将靶向蛋白质装载到新生成的外泌体中。已显示用载有蛋白质的EXPLORs处理可显著增加体内和体外的货物蛋白细胞内水平及其在受体细胞中的功能。这些结果清楚地表明，EXPLORs作为将基于蛋白质的治疗剂有效地细胞内转移到受体细胞和组织中的机制的潜力[127]。

4.2.7　装载的外泌体药物的靶向策略

诸多研究已成功证明药物可装载入外泌体中，形成的外泌体药物复合体递送至靶向组织或细胞中发挥作用。外泌体作为药物载体具有很好的稳定性和生物相容性，如何进行靶向策略的选择是将其应用于临床试验的必要环节。

将靶向肽添加到外泌体表面可以实现外泌体药物的靶向细胞识别。通过在供体细胞中过表达靶向肽使外泌体膜上带有该蛋白，分离外泌体后实现靶向识别，使外泌体内部装载治疗药物，且能靶向目标器官或细胞。许多类型的癌症中，表皮生长因子（epidermal growth factor receptor，EGFR）会过度表达和突变，EGFR变体Ⅲ型突变体（EGFRvⅢ）在许多肿瘤细胞比较常见，因此这两种受体都已被建议在许多癌症治疗环境中作为有效靶标[128]。日本东京医科大学（Tokyo Medical University）的Shin-ichiro Ohno等研究显示，外泌体可以有效地将miRNA传递到表达表皮生长因子受体（EGFR）的乳腺癌细胞[129]。他们通过改造供体细胞以表达融合至GE11肽的血小板衍生生长因子受体的跨膜结构域，可以实现靶向。他们的研究证明了外泌体携带的核酸药物能够靶向表达

EGFR的癌细胞。除了在外泌体膜上添加靶向肽实现靶向外，外泌体膜上还发现四跨膜结构蛋白，提示了外泌体来源和靶向信号选择的新可能。

外泌体药物的另一靶向策略是利用外泌体的归巢特性进行靶向识别。由于外泌体是由细胞分泌的囊泡，它们含有特定的脂质和细胞黏附分子，对受体细胞具有特异性。一些研究表明外泌体具有天然的靶向供体细胞的能力。MicroRNA（miRs）是多形胶质母细胞瘤（glioblastoma multiforme，GBM）的潜在治疗靶标，但不能准确的传递药物到肿瘤靶细胞阻碍了它们的广泛使用。间充质干细胞（Mesenchymal stem cells，MSC）可以迁移到包括GBM在内的癌症部位，并发挥抗肿瘤作用。伊朗德黑兰医科大学（Tehran University of Medical Sciences）的S. Sharif等研究发现脐带来源的间充质干细胞（Wharton's jelly-Mesenchymal stem cells，WJ-MSCs）分泌的外泌体能将标记的miRs-124传递至U87 GBM细胞中[130]。他们的研究表明，从WJ-MSC释放的外泌体传递外来miRNA，可能为GBM细胞瘤中miRNA替代疗法提供了新的可能。美国莱斯大学（Rice University）的Hongyun Zhao等研究发现成纤维细胞（Cancer-associated fibroblasts，CAFs）分泌的外泌体含有完整的代谢产物，包括氨基酸、脂质和三羧酸循环（tricarboxylic acid cycle，TCA）中间体，而癌细胞能摄取成纤维细胞衍生的外泌体来促进肿瘤生长[131]。2019年，研究人员综合了外泌体归巢特性与纳米药物的优势，利用肿瘤来源的外泌体构建了外泌体仿生多孔硅纳米颗粒作为靶向癌症化疗的药物载体[132]。这些研究表明，不同供体细胞衍生的外泌体可将药物递送至不同器官组织，但除了携带我们需要的靶向分子外，可能会携带其他与肿瘤发生、发展和转移的相关基因，在应用上仍存在一些潜在风险。

4.3　外泌体与疾病治疗

我国恶性肿瘤的发病率约占全球23.7%，死亡率约占全球30%[133]，已经成为威胁中国国民生活健康的主要原因。大多数肿瘤疾病由于其起病隐匿，病程演变快，使得很多肿瘤患者在初次诊断时就已经处于疾病晚期或已发生转移。当前应用相对广泛的肿瘤早期诊断方法主要包括组织活检、影像学检查等，但这些方法常具有创性、准确率低、特异性低等不足。因此，建立准确度高、特异性好的早期肿瘤诊断方法是预防肿瘤的重要方法之一。外泌体由于其特殊的生理形成过程和囊泡膜的保护作用，其内含物含量丰富、性质稳定，且其几乎存在于人体内所有部位，因此可应用于多种疾病的早期诊断，诊断指标的稳定性、检测的灵敏度、特异性都较现有临床开展的检验诊断指标有所提升。

近年来外泌体已成为肿瘤疾病研究中的热点，因其参与细胞间的通讯及遗传信息传递，对肿瘤疾病的发展有利有弊。不同来源的外泌体携带不同的蛋白质、核酸等细胞成分，其含有的蛋白质种类较多，如四次跨膜蛋白CD63、CD81、CD9，主要组织相容性复合物（Major histocompatibility complex，MHC）、热休克蛋白70（Heat shock protein，HSP70）及辅助蛋白Alix等。同时，外泌体还含有核酸如mRNA及miRNA等，介导细胞间的通讯及遗传信息的传递，并在多种疾病的诊断及预后中发挥着重要作用，如外泌体miR-150，miR-21，miR-192，let-7a，miR-223和miR-23a对结直肠癌源的诊断及预后判断有很高的价值，外泌体miR-126、miR-21可作为肺癌的诊断标志物等。由肿瘤细胞分泌的外泌体，可进入淋巴系统和肿瘤组织内的毛细血管，发挥对恶性肿瘤抑制或促进的双重调控作用[134]。外泌体能与肿瘤抑制因子相互作用，共同参与对肿瘤生长的调控。外泌体和p53细胞凋亡信号通路关系密切：一方面p53的许多靶基因，如TSAP6和CHMP4C等的转录激活促进外泌体形成；另一方面，外泌体分泌会外泄细胞内的p53，导致通过p53激活发挥作用的药物失效[135]。研究发现，外泌体能够将另一重要抑癌基因*PTEN*输送到靶细胞中，发挥其磷酸酶的活性，通过阻断促进细胞存活的Notch-1信号通路，抑制肿瘤细胞的增殖[136]。

人体内几乎所有细胞都可以分泌外泌体，无论是机体处于生理状态还是病理状态，我们均可从组织或体液中提取到一定量的外泌体，但对于同一组织或细胞而言，病理状态下的外泌体释放量常显著高于生理状态下。此外，由于外泌体特殊的生理形成过程，其内含物通常是来源于母细胞的蛋白分子、脂质、miRNAs、lncRNAs、circRNAs和DNA分子等，内含物的变化常常可以反映其来源母细胞中相应物质的变化情况。因此，近年来细胞外囊泡在许多疾病中的诊断作用越来越受到人们的关注。

microRNAs（miRNAs）是一类长度约为22nt、进化保守的非编码RNA分子，其参与基因表达的转录后调控。外泌体miRNAs可因脂质双分子层的保护作用而避免被降解，因此，其常常作为理想的体外循环分子诊断的标志物。目前，利用外泌体miRNAs作为疾病诊断标志物的研究陆续被报道。此外，外泌体囊泡内其他非编码RNAs或蛋白质分子也可在疾病的诊断中发挥重要作用[137]。

外泌体来源细胞可分为异常细胞和正常细胞，而目前具有治疗作用的外泌体主要是来源于正常细胞，其主要包括健康人体体细胞和干细胞两大类。干细胞可以通过旁分泌的形式来促进组织器官的修复，而外囊泡在旁分泌机制中发挥了重要的作用。外泌体可以通过携带干细胞来源的生物活性分子进入受体细胞而间接发挥干细胞的生物学功能，外泌体具有免疫原性低、相对易于管理、无致瘤性风险等优点。因此，近年来研究人员开始逐渐关注干细胞来源外泌体作为干细胞治疗的潜在替代品。干细胞来源的外泌体用于疾病治疗的报道也陆续发表，如干细胞来源的外泌体可用于皮肤损伤的修复；脂肪间充质干细胞来源的外泌体在体外可改善缺氧诱导的骨细胞凋亡和骨细胞介导的破骨细胞形成；干细胞、祖细胞来源的细胞外囊泡可用于治疗肾脏疾病；间充质干细胞来源的分泌体和细胞外囊泡用于放射性肺损伤的治疗；人脐带间充质干细胞来源的外泌体可通过降低巨噬细胞NLRP3炎症小体的活性来减轻急性肝衰竭；人肝脏干细胞来源的细胞外囊泡通过AKT-mTOR/PTEN联合调控增强肿瘤干细胞对酪氨酸激酶抑制剂的敏感性；间充质干细胞来源的细胞外囊泡可促进乳腺癌细胞的休眠，从而协助乳腺癌细胞治疗等[138]。其他来源于健康人体的非干细胞来源的外泌体也可用于疾病的治疗，如血小板微粒浸润实体肿瘤后通过转移mRNAs给受体细胞来抑制肿瘤生长，肝脏细胞来源外泌体也可用于病毒性肝炎、肝硬化和肝癌等的治疗[139]。

外泌体是细胞间信息交流的重要介质，其除了作为液体活检用于疾病的诊断外，在疾病治疗上也发挥了日益重要的作用。外泌体作为疾病治疗的方式主要包括两种，一种是直接携带其来源母细胞中物质进入受体细胞，来影响靶细胞功能；另一种是作为运载体将治疗性药物运输到靶器官或靶细胞，从而达到治疗目的。

外泌体可通过膜融合的方式进入靶细胞，由于其可以很自然地将核酸、蛋白质和脂质等物质传递给受体细胞，因此它们在靶向药物治疗的疾病领域中拥有很好的前景。相比于传统的靶向治疗药物运载体（如病毒、质粒），外泌体药物运载系统具有低免疫原性、高生物相容性、低毒性和可跨越血脑屏障等特征。目前，外泌体作为运载体用于靶向治疗的研究相对成熟，除了可以运输蛋白质和核酸（如miRNAs、lncRNAs），还可以运载中药物质等。外泌体作为载体在分子治疗中的应用广泛，如细胞外囊泡运载自杀性mRNA和/或蛋白用于恶性胶质瘤等恶性肿瘤的治疗；siGRP78修饰外泌体可使索拉非尼耐药的癌细胞对索拉非尼敏感[64]；外泌体运载的miRNA-142-3p抑制剂在体内外可降低乳腺癌的致瘤性；装载有siRNA外泌体可在体外传递到癌细胞中，并调控中细胞的增殖过程[139]。除此以外，外泌体也可运载治疗基因编辑工具或其他临床药物成分来达到疾病治疗的目的。

4.4　外泌体的应用和局限性

4.4.1　外泌体的主要应用

外泌体具有独特的组织或细胞特异性蛋白质和遗传物质，可反映其细胞来源和细胞的生理状态，因此，不同细胞的外泌体具有不同的特点和功能。探索不同细胞来源的外泌体的特点和功能有助于不同疾病的研究。除此之外，外泌体具有理想药物载体的许多特征。与一般外源性纳米载体相比，由于其内源性来源和表面功能性分子，在治疗神经退行性疾病方面显示出优越的治疗效果。

　　外泌体含有多种特异性蛋白质和核酸，具有作为天然载体的潜能。外泌体具有独特的生物活性，可作为小分子的载体被应用于治疗不同的疾病。在小鼠模型的试验中，外泌体可以携带难以跨越血脑屏障（blood-brain barrier，BBB）的姜黄素作用于小鼠上，可以使药物治疗活性维持稳定且能穿过血脑屏障，使小鼠免受脑炎症损害[140]。同时，外泌体还可以将阿霉素和紫杉醇运送至小鼠的肿瘤组织从而抑制肿瘤的生长。外泌体具有免受细胞吞噬的膜锚定蛋白与跨膜蛋白，能提高内容物的传递效率，内源性外泌体作为药物载体比使用合成纳米颗粒的细胞毒性效应要低，其逃脱吞噬清除的能力要比脂质体高。装载药物的外泌体的分子信号传导和药物的渗透及获取仍是试验上的挑战。

　　肿瘤来源的外泌体对抗肿瘤免疫也具有激活作用。外泌体能够将肿瘤特异性抗原，如MELAN-A，Silv，癌胚抗原（CEA）和间皮素等转移到树突状细胞，诱导CD8+T细胞介导的抗肿瘤免疫反应。在恶性脑胶质瘤患者体内，也存在类似由外泌体介导的针对自体肿瘤细胞的免疫反应。肿瘤细胞在应激后分泌的外泌体也会诱导特异性抗肿瘤反应，如热休克后淋巴瘤细胞释放的外泌体中MHC和共刺激分子水平持续增高，并诱导有效的抗肿瘤细胞免疫[141]。除了免疫激活效应，肿瘤外泌体还能直接诱导肿瘤细胞的凋亡。人胰腺癌细胞分泌的外泌体，使细胞内BCL相关的X（BCL2-Associated X，Bax）蛋白水平增加，而B淋巴细胞瘤-2（B-cell lymphoma-2，Bcl-2）的表达降低，促使肿瘤细胞进入线粒体凋亡途径；这些外泌体同时诱导PTEN磷酸酶和糖原合成酶激酶-3β（GSK-3β）的激活，降低细胞中丙酮酸脱氢酶的活性，抑制β-Catenin依赖信号和PI3K/AKT信号途径，促进肿瘤细胞凋亡途径；外泌体与胰腺癌细胞的相互作用还导致细胞核内Notch-1靶基因的表达下降，从而抑制Notch-1依赖的细胞存活途径[142]。外泌体其特有的优势在疾病的诊断、预防及治疗中仍有重要作用，相信在未来，外泌体会为临床肿瘤疾病诊断治疗提供更好的帮助。

　　尽管不断有报道发现肿瘤外泌体的潜在抗肿瘤作用，但对癌症晚期患者的研究中，更多的证据提示晚期肿瘤的外泌体反而抑制抗肿瘤的免疫应答，促进肿瘤的进展。带有Fas L和TRAIL等死亡配体的外泌体，使活化的T细胞出现凋亡；一些卵巢癌外泌体能够下调CD3ζ链的表达，抑制TCR信号和T细胞的功能；人乳腺癌和胸膜间皮瘤细胞系的外泌体含有NKG2D配体，能够抑制NK细胞和CD8+T细胞的细胞毒作用，促进肿瘤生长；人黑色素瘤细胞和大肠癌细胞分泌的外泌体则诱导单核细胞转化为免疫抑制细胞（MDSCs），由TGF-β1介导抑制T细胞的活性。

外泌体中的RNA和蛋白质参与对肿瘤侵袭和转移的调控。肿瘤细胞分泌的外泌体可通过其特定内容物（如TGF-β）介导经血液转移，同时促进成纤维细胞分化为成肌纤维细胞，减少Ⅰ型胶原的产生，增加金属基质蛋白酶（MMP）对胶原纤维的降解，从而促进肿瘤的转移[143]。缺氧多形性胶质瘤细胞来源的外泌体中的蛋白质和mRNA在肿瘤微血管形成中发挥重要作用。侵袭性胶质瘤细胞可通过外泌体向非侵袭性肿瘤细胞群转运突变EGFRvⅢ受体，受体细胞获得突变，激活细胞内MAPK和AKT信号通路，改变下游基因VEGF、Bcl-XL和p27的表达，进而获得侵袭性细胞表型[144]。此实验表明，外泌体能够改变肿瘤的侵袭表型。

外泌体中的mRNA和miRNA进入靶细胞后也可多形式调控肿瘤的进展。胶质瘤外泌体中的mRNA进入细胞后被翻译表达，刺激细胞增殖，促进肿瘤生长；转移性胃癌细胞来源的外泌体通过释放let-7家族的miRNA，拮抗其靶基因的抑癌作用，同时传递导致肿瘤转移的信号。外泌体还能参与肿瘤组织血管生成和表皮间充质转化（EMT）过程。相关研究表明，肿瘤外泌体可能通过调控VEGF和CXXCR4信号途径，增强血管生成和肿瘤生长能力；在EMT过程中，与肿瘤细胞间充质表型相关的基因表达增加，同时生成携带大量组织因子的外泌体，以维持适宜肿瘤生长的微环境，其具体机制尚在进一步研究中，外泌体还参与肿瘤细胞耐药性的产生[145]。肿瘤细胞还可通过外泌体排出化疗药物，并可中和基于抗体的靶向性药物。在耐药性人黑色素瘤细胞和卵巢癌细胞中均发现随着外泌体释放，细胞内药物浓度明显降低；而HER2分子，能够中和HER2抗体曲妥珠单抗，使作用于癌细胞的抗体减少，抑制疗效[146]。

关于外泌体的研究已经呈现出一些鲜明的特点。首先，绝大多数相关的研究视角是宏观和全息（holistic）的，更多的是从机体或细胞的功能和表型乃至疗效着眼，而并未对数量有限的特定基因进行过度解析。因此，长期以来深陷困惑和饱受挑战的中西医结合与中医药研究将在外泌体研究的背景下获得宝贵的启示和契机。外泌体不仅携带来源细胞的病理性或生理性标志蛋白或RNA，而其所含的活性分子则会直接具有药效作用，即外泌体本身可充当向特定病变部位转运药物、小分子或生物治疗、基因治疗制剂的载体，同时还具有被修饰、加工和改造的潜力。基于外泌体可以建立明确的肿瘤诊断方法，辅助肿瘤早期检测和诊断，帮助判断预后和治疗效果，并开发新的抗肿瘤药物和临床肿瘤干预措施。肿瘤来源外泌体的相关研究在某种程度上尤其体现出转化医学研究的思路和模式，将推动生物标志物研究进展，促进转化医学事业的进步。

4.4.2　外泌体对 CRISPR-Cas 系统的载运

基于CRISPR-Cas9系统的基因编辑技术已经在基础试验、医学研究和临床试验上被广泛地应用。尤其在临床应用上，如果能安全地将该系统传递到靶向组织和细胞，发挥其准确的剪切效果，定向的改变目标基因，在各种癌症、单基因和多基因遗传病，及病毒性疾病的治疗中将会有很大的突破。目前还没有一种安全且高效地传递载体用于CRISPR-Cas系统的体内运输。

来源于肿瘤细胞的外泌体可以借助自身的细胞嗜性高效靶向递送pCas9/sgRNA到肿瘤组织。韩国科学技术学院（Korea Institute of Science and Technology）的 Seung Min Kim等研究人员将载有CRIPSR-Cas9的肿瘤来源外泌体静脉注射到小鼠体内，实验发现该体系能够通过阻断多聚合酶-1（PARP-1）的基因表达，抑制肿瘤的生长[147]。内源性的外泌体或可用作CRISPR-Cas9系统一种安全有效的递送载体，但也可能使基因编辑技术的脱靶效应和安全性问题更加复杂。

由于外泌体尺寸较小，通过外泌体包装大分子核酸效率较低。中国中山大学的Lin Yao等将脂质体与外泌体融合形成外泌体-脂质体杂交纳米颗粒，能够有效地包裹大型质粒，也包括CRISPR-Cas9的表达载体，并靶向到间充质干细胞，被内吞后表达载体基因[148]。失活的Cas9（dCas9）mRNA的长度近5 000nt，难以通过电穿孔或其他方法封装到外泌体中。中国第四军医大学的

Li Zhelong等将外泌体膜蛋白CD9和人抗原R（HuR）融合，可对外泌体的RNA负载进行工程设计。他们在dCas9 mRNA序列中增加3个富AU原件（AU rich element，ARE），HuR是一种RNA结合蛋白，与RNA 序列中ARE具有高度亲和力，如此可将dCas9 mRNA和gRNA高效装载到CD9–HuR功能化的外泌体中。静脉给药后，CD9–HuR外泌体递送dCas9 mRNA和gRNA至肝脏，实现了基因沉默[149]。

4.4.3　外泌体在应用上的局限性

虽然外泌体在疾病的诊断治疗上具有很好的应用前景，大量的研究也证实了外泌体具有对外源分子的负载可能性以及成功递送至受体细胞的能力，但在临床应用试验之前仍要解决一些问题。首先，缺少标准化的提取方案，在本文中我们对常用以及新兴的提取方法优缺点进行了比较，随着外泌体应用的逐渐增多，我们必须开发出更统一、更简洁有效的标准化方法。其次，在对工程改造外泌体的加工和修饰过程中，供体细胞和外泌体的变化可能会影响蛋白质组成，这可能影响了工程化外泌体的生物活性和功效。因此，有必要选择对外泌体组成影响较小的方法和修饰过程中带来的细胞毒性等问题。最后，关于外泌体的生物安全性问题，外泌体在实现靶向治疗的过程中也可能将供体细胞来源的其他信息（如肿瘤发生、发展和转移的相关基因）带到靶向细胞、细胞中。因此，我们有必要充分了解外泌体产生机制和针对产生外泌体供体细胞的选择。尽管外泌体作为药物载体存在诸多挑战，但是纳米医学是一个快速发展的领域，相信会在不久的将来为现在面对的挑战提供解决方案。

在已知分泌外泌体的细胞类型中，人间充质干细胞是最有希望的细胞来源，但如何有效地分离和纯化外泌体仍然是一个巨大的挑战。目前，对于外泌体的主要提取方式是采用超速离心法，但这种方式获得的外泌体量很少，虽然也有其他提取方法，但都无法获得大量纯度高的外泌体，因此需要开发大规模生产，质量可控和快速纯化外泌体的技术平台。肿瘤来源的外泌体对肿瘤具有抑制或促进的双重作用，这可能是外泌体、细胞和环境因素之间复杂的相互作用的结果，与肿瘤进展程度和机体免疫状态密切相关。

5　RNA纳米颗粒修饰的外泌体作为CRISPR-Cas9系统的载体

许多对药物递送系统的研究中，由于完全分离各个种类的囊泡是不可能完成的，所以将外泌体和微囊统称为细胞外囊泡（extracellular vesicles，EVs）。外泌体即细胞外囊泡是一种由人体内各种类型的细胞所释放，并且含有RNA、脂质、蛋白质、代谢物以及其他分子的磷脂双层膜封闭的细胞间通讯结构，这些生物分子可以被各种类型的细胞分泌到生理液中。细胞外囊泡能够作为蛋白质、各种不同小分子和不同种类RNA的运送载体，将他们运送至受体细胞内部。外泌体作为载体可携带的核酸大分子有限。

美国辛辛那提大学（University of Cincinnati）的纳米领域杰出科学家郭培宣教授在*Nature Nanotechnology*杂志上发表文章，表明应用RNA纳米技术进行定向控制RNA纳米颗粒的优势[150-151]。此项技术用构建的抗体样RNA纳米颗粒修饰从HEK293T细胞培养上清液中纯化的细胞外囊泡，从而得到表面携带RNA纳米颗粒的细胞外囊泡，使相应的过度表达的受体癌细胞的靶向效率得到提高。作为测试疗法，文章中提及的细胞外囊泡都装载有用于下调生存素（Survivin）的小干扰RNA，生存素基因抑制细胞凋亡，并在许多癌症类型中过表达。将前列腺特异性膜抗原（PSMA）与携带抗体样RNA纳米颗粒的细胞外囊泡结合，以提高对前列腺癌细胞的靶向效率，抑制了小鼠前列腺癌的生长。乳腺癌细胞中因表皮生长因子受体（EGFR）过度表达，所以将表皮生长因子受体与携带抗体样RNA纳米颗粒的细胞外囊泡结合，抑制了小鼠乳腺癌的生长。同时，携带叶酸受体的细胞外囊泡也可以抑制结肠直肠肿瘤的生长。

　　抗体样RNA纳米颗粒可以实现RNA部分装载到细胞外囊泡或在细胞外囊泡表面修饰配体的机会。体外修饰方法使作为递送载体的细胞外囊泡的内源性成分得到了保留，就像构建其他合成纳米载体所需的那样，不需要在细胞外囊泡载体中构建人工内小体逃逸策略，就可用于siRNA的递送。在三种动物模型中，利用RNA配体的特异性靶向和细胞外囊泡的高效膜融合，显示配体的细胞外囊泡能够将siRNA特异性地运送到细胞内，增强了癌细胞特异性靶向，并有效地抑制了三种肿瘤的生长。特异性靶向癌细胞是将纳米囊泡应用于癌症治疗的重要前提，结果表明细胞外囊泡在体内具有生物相容性和良好的耐受性，没有观察到任何明显的毒性。

　　将抗体样（即Y形状）RNA纳米颗粒附着到微泡上，可以将有效的RNA治疗剂，如小分子干扰RNA（siRNA），特异性地递送给癌细胞。研究人员通过RNA纳米技术来应用RNA纳米颗粒并控制它们的去向，以产生能够在动物模型中成功靶向三种类型癌症的载有治疗剂的细胞外囊泡。该研究发现可促进使用siRNA、microRNA和其他RNA干扰技术的新一代抗癌药物的开发。

　　将有特殊结构的RNA（3WJ 结构，具有3 个端口，每个端口分别有不同作用：与靶头连接的靶向作用；与胆固醇配基相连的端口负责与外泌体连接；与荧光物质相连具有示踪作用。图5.1A和图5.2A）与外泌体相连，与不同的靶头相连即可靶向不同种类的癌细胞，经验证应用此系统作为载药传递系统能够体内外抑制多种癌细胞的生长。它们的组装原理示意图见图5.1B，我们用这种纳米颗粒修饰的外泌体包装了Survivin 的siRNA，在体外下调了survivin 基因的表达（图5.1C），在体内应用此技术抑制了前列腺癌和结肠癌细胞的生长（图5.1E、图5.2C和图5.2D）[150]。我们将利用此技术对本项目构建的Hypa-dcas9-HDAC1/gRNAKRAS 系统进行体内靶向转运。

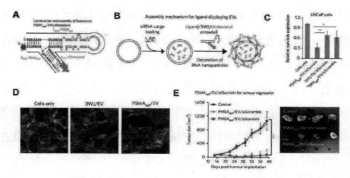

图 5.1　RNA 纳米颗粒修饰的外泌体结构和体内外抑制前列腺癌细胞生长

A—具有特殊结构RNA 构建示意图（PMSA适配体——红色，GFP——紫色，胆固醇配基——绿色）；B—RNA纳米颗粒修饰的外泌体载体系统组装示意图；C—qPCR实验表明载有Survivin siRNA的此载体系统可以抑制LNCap细胞中Survivin mRNA表达；D—RNA纳米颗粒修饰的外泌体在是否表达PSMA细胞中结合情况（细胞核—蓝色，细胞骨架—绿色，RNA纳米颗粒—红色）；E—载有Survivin siRNA 的RNA 纳米颗粒修饰的外泌体载体系统在裸鼠体内可以抑制肿瘤的生长。

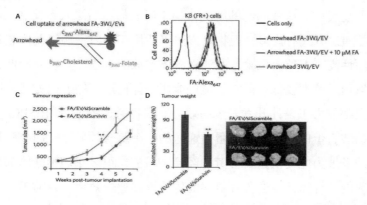

图 5.2　RNA 纳米颗粒修饰的外泌体结构和体内抑制结肠癌细胞生长

A—Floate-3WJ/EVs 组装示意图；B—Floate-3WJ/EVs 与具有叶酸受体（FR+）的KB细胞的结合情况；C—结肠癌裸鼠异种移植模型中，对照组和加药组分别尾静脉注射载有siR-Scramble 和siR-Survivin 的Floate-3WJ/EVs，6 周后与对照组相比，加药组荷瘤体积明显减小；D—结肠癌裸鼠异种移植模型中，对照组和加药组分别尾静脉注射载有siR-Scramble 和siR-Survivin 的Floate-3WJ/EVs，6 周后与对照组相比，加药组荷瘤重量明显减小。

纳米技术在生物应用上具有许多优点，该研究报道了应用RNA纳米技术方向的控制优势。改变箭头形状的RNA方向则可控制细胞外囊泡膜上的配体展示，或调节小干扰RNA（siRNA）或微小RNA（miRNA）的细胞内运输，使其具有特定的细胞靶向。在箭头的尾部放置膜锚定胆固醇，使其在细胞外囊泡的外表面上展示RNA适配体或叶酸，而将胆固醇置于箭头处会导致RNA纳米颗粒部分加载到细胞外囊泡中。利用特定靶向的RNA配体和细胞外囊泡进行有效的膜融合，得到的配体显示细胞外囊泡能够将siRNA特异的靶向细胞，并有效地阻断三种癌症模型中的肿瘤生长。基于RNA的疗法，如小干扰RNA，对于癌症治疗具有很大的希望，但是将这些药物递送至癌细胞中的靶标已经成为问题。总的来说，RNA纳米技术可以用来编程天然细胞外囊泡，特异性地将干扰RNA传递给癌细胞，向癌细胞提供有效的RNA治疗。研究人员正在努力将该技术应用到临床。

CRISPR-Cas9系统的出现简化了基因编辑的步骤，给基础研究和临床基因疾病、癌症治疗带来了便利和希望，但面临问题也有很多，如递送效率低、脱靶效应和免疫反应。这些问题的解决依赖于研究的不断深入和发展。CRISPR-Cas9系统的递送方式有许多，但物理方法不适用于体内；病毒载体装载能力有限、免疫原性高、有致癌风险；非病毒载体包载能力强，免疫原性低，且易于组装，虽然递送效率较低，但它是最可能用于体内给药的递送方式。因此，许多研究人员都致力于设计开发安全高效的非病毒递送系统。CRISPR-Cas9的递送本质是核酸、蛋白质或核糖核蛋白递送的一个综合领域，此前核酸和蛋白质递送载体的发展为此提供重要参考和经验。目前，很多非病毒载体都是基于不同类别材料的杂合体，综合各种材料的优势提高递送效率，目前阳离子脂质、阳离子聚合物、多肽、蛋白、金纳米粒、囊泡、金属材料和DNA纳米线团递送系统已经在体内、体外研究中取得了一系列进展。这些非病毒载体借助静电吸附、范德华力、氢键和共价键等装载CRISPR-Cas9系统，为适应全身给药，载体需要修饰PEG或包覆其他负电材料（如HA、环境响应性外壳）以增强载体循环稳定性。局部给药的基因编辑范围局限，安全性较好，不会引发大规模的脱靶效应，由于无须做到长循环，在体外层可以包覆PEI、PAsp（DET）等材料促进细胞摄取和内含体逃逸。CRISPR-Cas9技术具有广阔的应用前景，非病毒载体递送效率的不断提高必将助力CRISPR-Cas9技术的临床转化，为更多患者缓解甚至治愈疾病。

6 总结与展望

　　研究基因传递系统的一个重要目标是开发临床上可用于对抗癌症、艾滋病和阿尔茨海默氏病等难以捉摸的疾病的载体。如本章节所述，目前已经开发了各种各样的基因递送系统，并且许多都处在快速发展中，甚至临床试验中。但值得指出的是，尽管在过去的三十年中开发了许多病毒和非病毒基因递送系统，但是它们都具有一些缺点，使其在临床应用中仍有一定的局限性。有效改善当前可用系统的关键步骤包括：（1）改善细胞外靶向和递送；（2）增强细胞内递送和长时间表达；（3）减少对人体的毒性和副作用。

　　在过去的十年中，将外来体用作理想的递送系统引起了相当大的关注。这种天然载体在生物相容性和特异性，固有的长期循环能力，低毒性以及易于避免免疫系统识别和降低清除率等方面具有多方面的优势。考虑到所有这些因素，外泌体被认为是细胞或基因疗法的竞争性靶向递送载体，在多种疾病的治疗中具有多种优势和有希望的治疗价值。然而，其主要缺点是提取和分离过程效率低下，低的包封和装载效率，低的提取收率以及潜在地释放外来体中天然存在的不需要的物质。因此，需要在这一领域进行进一步研究，以标准化外泌体分离、纯化和储存的最佳方法。实际上，外泌体提取的几种方法劳动强度大，复杂且产率低，最近已开始通过使用一些有前景的技术（如磁吸附和流式细胞仪）以及诸如超声、电穿孔和孵育等装载技术来改善这一问题。然而，卸载外泌体的含量而不破坏结构完整性对于确保高的装载和包封效率都至关重要。总而言之，外泌体作为基因疗法的递送系统尚处于临床试验的早期阶段，但是由于该领域的研究发展非常迅速，希望在不久的将来可以攻克这些技术上的瓶颈，早日将其转移到临床和市场中。

参考文献

[1] ERIC S L. Initial impact of the sequencing of the human genome[J]. Nature, 2011, 470（7333）: 187–197.

[2] PAVLETICH P N, PABO C O. Zinc finger–DNA recognition: crystal structure of a Zif268–DNA complex at 2.1 A[J]. Science, 1991, 252（5007）: 809–817.

[3] TUPLER R, PERINI G, GREEN M R. Expressing the human genome[J]. Nature, 2001, 409（6822）: 832–833.

[4] BOCH J, SCHOLZE H, SCHORNACK S, et al. Breaking the code of DNA binding specificity of TAL–Type Ⅲ effectors[J]. Science, 2009, 326（5959）: 1509–1512.

[5] MAK N S, BRADLEY P, CERNADAS R A, et al. The crystal structure of TAL effector PthXo1 bound to its DNA target[J]. Science, 2012, 335（6069）: 716–719.

[6] JINEK, MARTIN, CHYLINSKI, et al. A programmable Dual–RNA–Guided DNA endonuclease in adaptive bacterial immunity[J]. Science, 2012, 337（6096）: 816–821.

[7] CONG L, RAN F A, COX D, et al. Multiplex genome engineering using CRISPR/Cas systems[J]. Science, 2013, 339（6121）: 819–823.

[8] KOMOR A C, KIM Y B, PACKER M S, et al. Programmable editing of a target base in genomic DNA without double–stranded DNA cleavage[J]. Nature, 2016, 533（7603）: 420–424.

[9] GAUDELLI N M, KOMOR A C, REES H A, et al. Programmable base editing of A•T to G•C in genomic DNA without DNA cleavage[J]. Nature, 2017, 551（11）: 464–471.

[10] LINO C A, HARPER J C, CARNEY J P, et al. Delivering CRISPR: a review of the challenges and approaches[J]. Drug Delivery, 2018, 25（1）: 1234–1257.

[11] YIN H, KAUFFMAN K J, ANDERSON D G. Delivery technologies for genome editing[J]. Nature Reviews Drug Discovery, 2017, 16（6）: 387–399.

[12] LIU C, ZHANG L, LIU H, et al. Delivery strategies of the CRISPR–Cas9 gene–editing system for therapeutic applications[J]. Journal of Controlled Release, 2017, 266: 17–26.

[13] LI H, YANG Y, HONG W, et al. Applications of genome editing technology in the targeted therapy of human diseases: mechanisms, advances and prospects[J]. Signal Transduction and Targeted Therapy, 2020, 5（1）: 1.

[14] KOTTERMAN M A, SCHAFFER D V. Engineering adeno–associated viruses for clinical gene therapy[J]. Nature Reviews Genetics, 2014, 15（7）: 445–451.

[15] MAGGIO I, HOLKERS M, LIU J, et al. Adenoviral vector delivery of RNA–guided CRISPR/Cas9 nuclease complexes induces targeted mutagenesis in a diverse array of human cells[J]. Scientific Reports, 2014, 4（1）: 5105.

[16] PAULK N K, WURSTHORN K, WANG Z, et al. Adeno–ssociated virus gene repair corrects a mouse model of hereditary tyrosinemia in vivo[J]. Hepatology. 2010, 51（4）: 1200–1208.

[17] KOIKE–YUSA H, LI Y, TAN E P, et al. Genome–wide recessive genetic screening in mammalian cells with a lentiviral CRISPR–guide RNA library[J]. Nature Biotechnology, 2013, 32（3）: 267–273.

[18] ANSON D S. The use of retroviral vectors for gene therapy–what are the risks? A review of retroviral pathogenesis and its relevance to retroviral vector–mediated gene delivery[J]. Genetic vaccines and therapy, 2004, 2（1）: 9.

[19] STOYE J P, COFFIN J M. The four classes of endogenous murine leukemia virus: structural relationships and potential for recombination[J]. Journal of Virology, 1987, 61（9）: 2659.

[20] XU Y, ZHENHUA Z, LIXIN G, et al. BMP7overexpressing bone marrowderived mesenchymal stem cells（BMSCs）are more effective than wildtype BMSCs in healing fractures[J]. Experimental & Therapeutic Medicine, 2018, 16（2）: 1381–1388.

[21] NIU D, WEI H J, LIN L, et al. Inactivation of porcine endogenous retrovirus in pigs using CRISPR–Cas9[J]. Science, 2017, 357（6357）: 1303.

[22] DAVID, ESCORSKARINE, BRECKPOT. Lentiviral vectors in gene therapy: Their current status and future potential[J]. Archivum Immunologiae et Therapiae Experimentalis, 2010, 58: 107–119.

[23] ZUFFEREY R, DULL T, MANDEL R J, et al. Self–inactivating lentivirus vector for safe and efficient in vivo gene delivery[J]. Journal of virology, 1998, 72（12）: 9873–9880.

[24] SCHNELL T, FOLEY P, WIRTH M, et al. Development of a self–inactivating, minimal

lentivirus vector based on simian immunodeficiency virus[J]. Human Gene Therapy, 2000, 11（3）: 439-447.

[25] CONNOLLY, J B. Lentiviruses in gene therapy clinical research[J]. Gene Therapy, 2002, 9（24）: 1730-1734.

[26] AMAZIAH, COLEMAN, JAMES E, et al. Lentiviral hematopoietic stem cell gene therapy in patients with wiskott-Aldrich syndrome[J]. Science, 2013, 341（6148）: 1233151.

[27] CARTIER N, HACEIN-BEY-ABINA S, BARTHOLOMAE C, et al. Hematopoietic stem cell gene therapy with a lentiviral vector in X-linked adrenoleukodystrophy[J]. Science, 2009, 326（5954）: 818-823.

[28] FEI Z, WU X P, LEI W, et al. Role of FGF-2 transfected bone marrow mesenchymal stem cells in engineered bone tissue for repair of avascular necrosis of femoral head in rabbits[J]. Cellular Physiology and Biochemistry, 2018, 48（2）: 773-784.

[29] TEBAS P, STEIN D, TANG W W, et al. Gene editing of CCR5 in autologous CD4 T cells of persons infected with HIV[J]. New England Journal of Medicine, 2014, 370（10）: 901-910.

[30] BANK A, DORAZIO R, LEBOULCH P. A phase I / II clinical trial of beta-globin gene therapy for beta-thalassemia[J]. Annals of the New York Academy of Sciences, 2005, 1054（1）: 308-316.

[31] NANOU A, AZZOUZ M. Gene therapy for neurodegenerative diseases based on lentiviral vectors[J]. Progress in Brain Research, 2009, 175（175）: 187-200.

[32] PALFI S, GURRUCHAGA J M, RALPH G S, et al. Long-term safety and tolerability of ProSavin, a lentiviral vector-based gene therapy for Parkinson's disease: a dose escalation, open-label, phase 1/2 trial[J]. Lancet, 2014, 383（9923）: 1138-1146.

[33] FABRIZIA U, BEATRIZ C F, MASIUK K E, et al. Gene therapy for sickle cell disease: A lentiviral vector comparison study[J]. Human gene therapy, 2018, 29（10）: 1153-1166.

[34] MILONE M C, O'DOHERTY U. Clinical use of lentiviral vectors[J]. Leukemia Official Journal of the Leukemia Society of America Leukemia Research Fund U K, 2018, 32（15）: 1529-1541.

[35] BURNS J C, FRIEDMANN T, DRIEVER W, et al. Vesicular stomatitis virus G glycoprotein pseudotyped retroviral vectors: concentration to very high titer and efficient gene transfer into mammalian and nonmammalian cells[J]. Proceedings of the National Academy of Sciences, 1993, 90（17）: 8033-8037.

[36] ROWE W P, HUEBNER R J, GILMORE L K, et al. Isolation of a cytopathogenic agent from human adenoids undergoing spontaneous degeneration in tissue culture[J]. Proc Soc Exp Biol

Med, 1953, 84（3）: 570–573.

[37] DHINGRA A, HAGE E, GANZENMUELLER T, et al. Molecular evolution of human adenovirus（HAdV）species C[J]. Scientific Reports, 2019, 9（9）: 441–462.

[38] KING A M Q, ADAMS M J, GARSTENS E B, et al. Virus taxonomy: ninth report of the international committee on taxonomy of viruses[J]. Portland, 2012, 27（6）.

[39] A G G, B C R B, C D M L, et al. Genomic characterization of human adenovirus type 4 strains isolated worldwide since 1953 identifies two separable phylogroups evolving at different rates from their most recent common ancestor[J]. Virology, 2019, 538: 11–23.

[40] ROBINSON C M, SINGH G, LEE J Y, et al. Molecular evolution of human adenoviruses[J]. Scientific Reports, 2013, 3（1）: 1812.

[41] CRENSHAW B J, JONES L B, BELL C R, et al. Perspective on adenoviruses: Epidemiology, pathogenicity, and gene therapy[J]. Biomedicines, 2019, 7（3）: 61.

[42] C C S L A B, B E S B, D R Z C, et al. Adenovirus–mediated gene delivery: Potential applications for gene and cell–based therapies in the new era of personalized medicine[J]. Genes & Diseases, 2017, 4（2）: 43–63.

[43] TOTH K, WOLD W S M. Adenovirus vectors for gene therapy, vaccination and cancer gene therapy[J]. Current Gene Therapy, 2013, 13（6）: 421–433.

[44] GINN S L, AMAYA A K, ALEXANDER I E, et al. Gene therapy clinical trials worldwide to 2017: An update[J]. The Journal of Gene Medicine, 2018, 20（5）.

[45] JAFFE H A, DANEL C, LONGENECKER G, et al. Adenovirus–mediated in vivo gene transfer and expression in normal rat liver[J]. Nature Genetics, 1992, 1（5）: 372–378.

[46] YIZHE T, HONGJU W, HIDEYO U, et al. Derivation of a triple mosaic adenovirus for cancer gene therapy[J]. PLOS ONE, 2009, 4（12）: 8526.

[47] ANURAG S, MANISH T, DINESH S B, et al. Adenoviral vector–based strategies for cancer therapy[J]. Curr Drug Ther, 2009, 4（2）: 117–138.

[48] ZHANG W W, LI L J, LI D G, et al. The first approved gene therapy product for cancer Ad–p53（Gendicine）: 12 years in the clinic[J]. Human Gene Therapy, 2018, 29（2）: 160–179.

[49] MARASINI S, CHANG D Y, JUNG J H, et al. Effects of adenoviral gene transduction on the stemness of human bone marrow mesenchymal stem cells[J]. Molecules & Cells, 2017, 40(8): 598–605.

[50] B S P B A, D M E C, E C D, et al. Use of adenovirus type–5 vectored vaccines: a cautionary

tale[J]. Lancet, 2020, 396 (10260): 68–69.

[51] WILLIAMS P D, RANJZAD P, KAKAR S J, et al. Development of viral vectors for use in cardiovascular gene therapy[J]. Viruses, 2010, 2 (2): 334–371.

[52] JEYANATHAN M, THANTHRIGE–DON N, AFKHAMI S, et al. Novel chimpanzee adenovirus–vectored respiratory mucosal tuberculosis vaccine: overcoming local anti–human adenovirus immunity for potent TB protection[J]. Mucosal Immunology, 2015, 8 (6): 1373–1387.

[53] ATCHISON R W, CASTO B C, HAMMON W M. Adenovirus–associated defective virus particles[J]. Science, 1965, 149 (3685): 754–755.

[54] SONNTAG F, SCHMIDT K, KLEINSCHMIDT J A. A viral assembly factor promotes AAV2 capsid formation in the nucleolus[J]. Proceedings of the National Academy of Sciences of the United States of America, 2010, 107 (22): 10220–10225.

[55] PAULK N K, WURSTHORN K, WANG Z, et al. Adeno–associated virus gene repair corrects a mouse model of hereditary tyrosinemia in vivo[J]. Hepatology, 2010, 51 (4): 1200–1208.

[56] GAJ T, EPSTEIN B E, SCHAFFER D V. Genome engineering using adeno–associated virus: basic and clinical research applications[J]. Molecular Therapy the Journal of the American Society of Gene Therapy, 2016, 24 (3) 458–464.

[57] GRIMM D, LEE J S, WANG L, et al. In vitro and in vivo gene therapy vector evolution via multispecies interbreeding and retargeting of adeno–associated viruses[J]. Journal of Virology, 2008, 82 (12): 5887–5911.

[58] GRIMM D, KAY M A, From virus evolution to vector revolution: use of naturally occurring serotypes of adeno–associated virus (AAV) as novel vectors for human gene therapy[J]. Current Gene Therapy, 2003, 3 (4): 281–304.

[59] SEPPO, YLÄ–HERTTUALA. Endgame: Glybera finally recommended for approval as the first gene therapy drug in the european union[J]. Molecular Therapy the Journal of the American Society of Gene Therapy, 2012, 20 (10): 1831–1832.

[60] LIU C, ZHANG L, LIU H, et al. Delivery strategies of the CRISPR–Cas9 gene–editing system for therapeutic applications[J]. Journal of Controlled Release, 2017: 17–26.

[61] CONG L, RAN F A, COX D, et al. Multiplex genome engineering using CRISPR/Cas Systems[J]. science, 2013, 339 (6121): 819–823.

[62] ANN F, RAN, CONG, et al. In vivo genome editing using staphylococcus aureus Cas9[J]. Nature, 2015, 520 (7546): 186–191.

[63] FRIEDLAND A E, BARAL R, SINGHAL P, et al. Characterization of staphylococcus aureus Cas9: A smaller Cas9 for all-in-one adeno-associated virus delivery and paired nickase applications[J]. Genome biology, 2015, 16 (1): 1-10.

[64] SWIECH L, HEIDENREICH M, BANERJEE A, et al. In vivo interrogation of gene function in the mammalian brain using CRISPR-Cas9[J]. Nature Biotechnology, 2015, 33 (1): 102-106.

[65] YANG Y, WANG L, BELL P, et al. A dual AAV system enables the Cas9-mediated correction of a metabolic liver disease in newborn mice[J]. Nature Biotechnology, 2016, 34 (3): 334-338.

[66] ZETSCHE B, VOLZ S E, ZHANG F. A split-Cas9 architecture for inducible genome editing and transcription modulation[J]. Nature Biotechnology, 2015, 33 (2): 139-142.

[67] BERNS K I, DAYA S. Gene Therapy using adeno-associated virus vectors[J]. Clinical Microbiology Reviews, 2008, 21 (4): 583-593.

[68] LHERITEAU E, DAVIDOFF A M, NATHWANI A C. Haemophilia gene therapy: Progress and challenges[J]. Blood Reviews, 2015, 29 (5): 321-328.

[69] NATHWANI A C, REISS U M, TUDDENHAM E G D, et al. Long-term safety and efficacy of factor IX gene therapy in hemophilia B[J]. New England Journal of Medicine, 2014, 371 (21): 1994-2004.

[70] WEBER N D, DANIEL S, HALL S R, et al. AAV-mediated delivery of zinc finger nucleases targeting hepatitis B virus inhibits active replication[J]. Plos One, 2014, 9 (5): 97579.

[71] TSENG W S, CHEN C, BRESLIN M B, et al. Tumor-specific promoter-driven adenoviral therapy for insulinoma[J]. Cellular Oncology, 2016, 39 (3): 279-286.

[72] PERABO L, GOLDNAU D, WHITE K, et al. Heparan sulfate proteoglycan binding properties of adeno-associated virus retargeting mutants and consequences for their in vivo tropism[J]. Journal of Virology, 2006, 80 (14): 7265.

[73] HILDINGER M, AURICCHIO A. Advances in AAV-mediated gene transfer for the treatment of inherited disorders[J]. European Journal of Human Genetics Ejhg, 2004, 12 (4): 263.

[74] YIN H, KANASTY R L, ELTOUKHY A A, et al. Non-viral vectors for gene-based therapy[J]. Nature Reviews Genetics, 2014, 15 (8): 541-555.

[75] GU Z, BISWAS A, ZHAO M, et al. Tailoring nanocarriers for intracellular protein delivery[J]. Cheminform, 2011, 40 (7): 3638-3655.

[76] DAN P, KARP J M, HONG S, et al. Nanocarriers as an emerging platform for cancer therapy[J]. Nature nanotechnology, 2007, 2 (12): 751-760.

[77] MATSUMURA Y, MAEDA H. A new concept for macromolecular therapeutics in cancer chemotherapy: Mechanism of tumoritropic accumulation of proteins and the antitumor agent smancs[J]. Cancer Research, 1986, 46 (12 Pt 1): 6387–6392.

[78] FROKJAER S, OTZEN D E. Protein drug stability: a formulation challenge[J]. Nature Reviews Drug Discovery, 2005, 4 (4): 298–306.

[79] JAMES N D, COKER R J, TOMLINSON D, et al. Liposomal doxorubicin (Doxil): An effective new treatment for Kaposi's sarcoma in AIDS[J]. Clinical Oncology, 1994, 6 (5): 294–296.

[80] SARA S, JOÃO S, ALBERTO P, et al. Nanomedicine: Principles, properties, and regulatory issues[J]. Frontiers in Chemistry, 2018, 20 (6): 360.

[81] PATRA J K, DAS G, FRACETO L F, et al. Nano based drug delivery systems: recent developments and future prospects[J]. Journal of Nanobiotechnology, 2018, 16 (1): 71.

[82] SINGH A P, BISWAS A, SHUKLA A, et al. Targeted therapy in chronic diseases using nanomaterial–based drug delivery vehicles[J]. Signal Transduction and Targeted Therapy, 2019, 4 (1): 33.

[83] GARIBAY A P R D, SOLINÍS M A, POZO-RODRÍGUEZ A D, et al. Solid lipid nanoparticles as non–viral vectors for gene transfection in a cell model of fabry disease[J]. Journal of Biomedical Nanotechnology, 2015, 11 (3): 500.

[84] JOSUNE, TORRECILLA, ANA, et al. Solid lipid nanoparticles as non–viral vector for the treatment of chronic hepatitis C by RNA interference[J]. International Journal of Pharmaceutics, 2015, 479 (1): 181–188.

[85] TORRECILLA J, POZO-RODRÍGUEZ D A, SOLINÍS M Á, et al. Silencing of hepatitis C virus replication by a non–viral vector based on solid lipid nanoparticles containing a shRNA targeted to the internal ribosome entry site (IRES)[J]. Colloids & Surfaces B Biointerfaces, 2016, 146: 808–817.

[86] POZO-RODRÍGUEZ A D, DELGADO D, SOLINÍS M Á, et al. Solid lipid nanoparticles as potential tools for gene therapy: in vivo protein expression after intravenous administration[J]. International Journal of Pharmaceutics, 2010, 385 (1–2): 157–162.

[87] BATTAGLIA L, SERPE L, FOGLIETTA F, et al. Application of lipid nanoparticles to ocular drug delivery[J]. Expert Opinion on Drug Delivery, 2016, 13 (12): 1743–1757.

[88] DEL POZO-RODRÍGUEZ, ANA, ÁNGELES SOLINÍS, MARÍA, RODRÍGUEZ-GASCÓN, ALICIA. Applications of lipid nanoparticles in gene therapy[J]. European Journal

of Pharmaceutics and Biopharmaceutics，2016，109：184-193.

[89] MALI P，AACH J，STRANGES P B，et al. CAS9 transcriptional activators for target specificity screening and paired nickases for cooperative genome engineering，2013，31（9）：833-838.

[90] RAGHAVAN A，et al. High-throughput screening and CRISPR-Cas9 modeling of causal lipid-associated expression quantitative trait locus variants[J]. bioRxiv，2016，056820.

[91] PLATT R J，CHEN S D，ZHOU Y，et al. CRISPR-Cas9 knockin mice for genome editing and cancer modeling[J]. Cell，2014，159（2）：440-455.

[92] YIN H，SONG C Q，DORKIN J R，et al. Therapeutic genome editing by combined viral and non-viral delivery of CRISPR system components in vivo[J]. Nature Biotechnology，2016，34（3）：328-333.

[93] ZURIS J A，THOMPSON D B，SHU Y，et al. Cationic lipid-mediated delivery of proteins enables efficient protein-based genome editing in vitro and in vivo[J]. Nature Biotechnology，2015.

[94] WANG M，ZURIS J A，MENG F，et al. Efficient delivery of genome-editing proteins using bioreducible lipid nanoparticles[J]. Proc Natl Acad Sci U S A，2016，113（11）：2868-2873.

[95] HORII T，TAMURA D，MORITA S，et al. Generation of an ICF syndrome model by efficient genome editing of human induced pluripotent stem cells using the CRISPR system[J]. International Journal of Molecular Sciences，2013，14（10）：19774-19781.

[96] SAKUMA T，NISHIKAWA A，KUME S，et al. Multiplex genome engineering in human cells using all-in-one CRISPR/Cas9 vector system[J]. Scientific Reports，2014，4：5400.

[97] MILLER JB，ZHANG S，KOS P，et al. Non-viral CRISPR/Cas gene editing in vitro and in vivo enabled by synthetic nanoparticle co-delivery of Cas9 mRNA and sgRNA[J]. Angew Chem Int Ed Engl，2017，56（4）：1059-1063.

[98] LIU J，CHANG J，JIANG Y，et al. Fast and efficient CRISPR/Cas9 genome editing in vivo enabled by bioreducible lipid and messenger RNA nanoparticles[J]. Advanced Materials，2019，31（33）.

[99] ZHANG X，LI B，LUO X，et al. Biodegradable amino-ester nanomaterials for Cas9 mRNA delivery in vitro and in vivo[J]. Acs Applied Materials & Interfaces，2017，9（30）：25481.

[100] FINN J D，SMITH A R，PATEL M C，et al. A single administration of CRISPR/Cas9 lipid nanoparticles achieves robust and persistent invivo genome editing[J]. Cell Reports，2018，22（9）：2227-2235.

[101] BOBO D，ROBINSON KJ，ISLAM J，et al. Nanoparticle-based medicines：a review of

FDA-approved materials and clinical trials to date[J]. Pharm Res, 2016, 33 (10):
2373-2387.

[102] Celator Pharmaceuticals, Inc. Celator announces phase 3 trial for VYXEOSTM (CPX-
351) in patients with high-risk acute myeloid leukemia demonstrates statistically significant
improvement in overall survival[J]. Biotech Week, 2016.

[103] 柯刚, 伍振峰, 杨明, 等. 脂质体技术的转化应用分析及关键问题研究 [J]. 世界中医药,
2015 (03): 35-40.

[104] XIANG X Y, DU S, DING Y, et al. Application and development of liposome injection[J].
China Pharm Univ, 2020, 51 (4): 383-393.

[105] MALLICK S, CHOI J S. Liposomes: Versatile and biocompatible nanovesicles for efficient
biomolecules delivery[J]. Journal of Nanoscience and Nanotechnology, 2014, 14 (1): 755-765.

[106] JOHNSTONE R M, ADAM M, HAMMOND J R, et al. Vesicle formation during reticulocyte
maturation. Association of plasma membrane activities with released vesicles (exosomes) [J].
The Journal of biological chemistry, 1987, 262 (19): 9412-9420.

[107] THÉRY C, ZITVOGEL L, AMIGORENA S. Exosomes: composition, biogenesis and
function[J]. Nature Reviews Immunology, 2002, 2 (8): 569-579.

[108] CAROLINA D L T G, GOREHAM R V, BECH S J J, et al. "Exosomics" —A review of
biophysics, biology and biochemistry of exosomes with a focus on human breast milk[J].
Frontiers in Genetics, 2018, 9: 92.

[109] 蒋航, 陈波, 曾雪, 等. 外泌体在胶质瘤中的研究进展 [J]. 中国肿瘤, 2020, 29 (10):
777-786.

[110] 陈文生, 赵颖海. 外泌体提取方法及其在人类疾病中的研究进展 [J]. 海南医学,
2019, 30 (22): 2977-2980.

[111] 寿崟, 马宇航, 虎力, 等. 外泌体研究在中医学领域的应用及前景 [J]. 上海中医药大
学学报, 2019, 33 (06): 38-43.

[112] 李双双, 杜春阳, 袁媛, 等. 不同细胞来源的外泌体的特点和功能 [J]. 国际药学研究
杂志, 2019, 46 (06): 411-417.

[113] 吴忧, 辛林. 新的药物传递系统: 外泌体作为药物载体递送 [J]. 中国生物工程杂志,
2020, 40 (09): 28-35.

[114] 周建芬, 柴芝兰, 谢操, 等. 外泌体作为药物递送载体的研究进展 [J]. 中国医药工业
杂志, 2020, 51 (04): 425-433.

[115] SUN D, ZHUANG X, XIANG X, et al. A novel nanoparticle drug delivery system: the anti-inflammatory activity of curcumin is enhanced when encapsulated in exosomes[J]. Mol Ther, 2010, 18（9）: 1606–1614.

[116] AGRAWAL A K, AQIL F, JEYABALAN J, et al. Milk-derived exosomes for oral delivery of paclitaxel[J]. Nanomedicine Nanotechnology Biology & Medicine, 2017, 13（5）: 1627–1636.

[117] ALVAREZ-ERVITI L, SEOW Y, YIN H F, et al. Delivery of siRNA to the mouse brain by systemic injection of targeted exosomes[J]. Nature Biotechnology, 2011, 29（4）: 341.

[118] HOOD J L, SCOTT M J, WICKLINE S A, Maximizing exosome colloidal stability following electroporation[J]. Analytical Biochemistry, 2014, 448（1）: 41–49.

[119] LAMICHHANE T N, RAIKER R S, JAY S M. Exogenous DNA loading into extracellular vesicles via electroporation is size-dependent and enables limited gene delivery[J]. Mol Pharm, 2015, 12（10）: 3650–3657.

[120] KOOIJMANS S A A, STREMERSCH S, BRAECKMANS K, et al. Electroporation-induced siRNA precipitation obscures the efficiency of siRNA loading into extracellular vesicles[J]. Journal of Controlled Release, 2013, 172（1）: 229–238.

[121] SHTAM T A, KOVALEV R A, VARFOLOMEEVA E Y, et al. Exosomes are natural carriers of exogenous siRNA to human cells in vitro[J]. Cell Communication & Signaling, 2013, 11(1):88.

[122] FAMILTSEVA A, JEREMIC N, TYAGI S C. Exosomes: cell-created drug delivery systems[J]. Molecular and Cellular Biochemistry, 2019, 459（1–2）: 1–6.

[123] LV L H, WAN Y L, LIN Y, et al. Anticancer drugs cause release of exosomes with heat shock proteins from human hepatocellular carcinoma cells that elicit effective natural killer cell antitumor responses in vitro [J]. Journal of Biological Chemistry, 2012, 287（19）: 15874–15885.

[124] LAVINIA R, ANGELA D L, NICOLA A, et al. Involvement of multiple myeloma cell-derived exosomes in osteoclast differentiation[J]. Oncotarget, 2015, 6（15）: 13772–13789.

[125] WANG H, SUN H J, ZHENG Y, et al. Curcumin-primed exosomes potently ameliorate cognitive function in AD mice by inhibiting hyperphosphorylation of the Tau protein through the AKT/GSK-3 β pathway[J]. Nanoscale, 2019, 11（15）: 7481–7496.

[126] ZHANG H, BAI M, DENG T, et al. Cell-derived microvesicles mediate the delivery of miR-29a/c to suppress angiogenesis in gastric carcinoma[J]. Cancer Letters, 2016, 375（2）: 331–339.

[127] YIM N, RYU S W, CHOI K, et al. Exosome engineering for efficient intracellular delivery of soluble proteins using optically reversible protein-protein interaction module[J]. Nature

Communications，2016，7（1）：12277.

[128] NEDERGAARD M K，HEDEGAARD C J，POULSEN H S. Targeting the epidermal growth factor receptor in solid tumor malignancies[J]. Biodrugs Clinical Immunotherapeutics Biopharmaceuticals & Gene Therapy，2012，26（2）：83-99.

[129] OHNO S I，TAKANASHI M，SUDO K，et al. Systemically injected exosomes targeted to EGFR deliver antitumor microRNA to breast cancer cells[J]. Molecular therapy：the journal of the American Society of Gene Therapy，2013，21（1）：185-191.

[130] SHARIF S，GHAHREMANI M H，SOLEIMANI M. Delivery of exogenous miR-124 to glioblastoma multiform cells by wharton's jelly mesenchymal stem cells decreases cell proliferation and migration，and confers chemosensitivity[J]. Stem Cell Reviews & Reports，2018，14（10）：236-246.

[131] ZHAO H Y，YANG L F，JOELLE B，et al. Tumor microenvironment derived exosomes pleiotropically modulate cancer cell metabolism[J]. eLife.，2016，5：10250.

[132] YONG T，ZHANG X，BIE N，et al. Tumor exosome-based nanoparticles are efficient drug carriers for chemotherapy[J]. Nature Communications，2019，10（1）：751-760.

[133] Global cancer observatory：cancer today

[134] 崔国宁，刘喜平，虎峻瑞，等. 不同来源外泌体与肿瘤发病相关性的研究与进展[J]. 中国组织工程研究，2020，24（13）：2095-2101.

[135] YU X，RILEY T，LEVINE A J. The regulation of the endosomal compartment by p53 the tumor suppressor gene[J]. Febs Journal，2010，276（8）：2201-2212.

[136] Putz U，Howitt J，Doan A，et al. The tumor suppressor PTEN is exported in exosomes and has phosphatase activity in recipient cells[J]. Science Signaling，2012，5（243）：70.

[137] 陈洁，程福，黄远帅，等. 外泌体在疾病诊疗中的研究进展[J]. 标记免疫分析与临床，2019，26（11）：1972-1976.

[138] PHINNEY D G，PITTENGER M F. Concise review：MSC-derived exosomes for cell-free therapy[J]. Stem cells，2017，35（4）：851-858.

[139] LI Y，ZHANG Y，LI Z，et al. Exosomes as carriers for anti-tumor therapy[J]. ACS Biomaterials Science and Engineering，2019，5（10），4870-4881.

[140] CHEN W，WANG J，SHAO C，et al. Efficient induction of antitumor T cell immunity by exosomes derived from heat-shocked lymphoma cells[J]. European Journal of Immunology，2010，36（6）：1598-1607.

[141] AZMI A S, BAO B, SARKAR F H. Exosomes in cancer development, metastasis, and drug resistance: a comprehensive review[J]. Cancer & Metastasis Reviews, 2013, 32(3-4): 623-642.

[142] IERO M, VALENTI R, HUBER V, et al. Tumour-released exosomes and their implications in cancer immunity[J]. Cell Death & Differentiation, 2008, 15(1): 80-88.

[143] AL-NEDAWI K, MEEHAN B, MICALLEF J, et al. Intercellular transfer of the oncogenic receptor EGFRvIII by microvesicles derived from tumour cells[J]. Nature cell biology, 2008, 10(5): 619-624.

[144] MASHOURI L, YOUSEFI H, AREF A R, et al. Exosomes: composition, biogenesis, and mechanisms in cancer metastasis and drug resistance[J]. Molecular Cancer, 2019, 18(1): 75.

[145] MARTINEZ VG, O'NEILL S, SALIMU J, et al. Resistance to HER2-targeted anti-cancer drugs is associated with immune evasion in cancer cells and their derived extracellular vesicles[J]. Oncoimmunology, 2017, 6(12): 1362530.

[146] SEUNG M K, YOOSOO Y, SEUNG J O, et al. Cancer-derived exosomes as a delivery platform of CRISPR/Cas9 confer cancer cell tropism-dependent targeting – ScienceDirect[J]. Journal of Controlled Release, 2017, 266(28): 8-16.

[147] LIN Y, WU J, GU W, et al. Exosome - liposome hybrid nanoparticles deliver CRISPR/Cas9 system in MSCs[J]. Advanced Science, 2018, 5(4): 1700611.

[148] LI Z, ZHOU X, WEI M, et al. In vitro and in vivo RNA inhibition by CD9-HuR functionalized exosomes encapsulated with miRNA or CRISPR/dCas9[J]. Nano Letters, 2018, 19(1): 19-28.

[149] PI F, BINZEL D W, LEE T J, et al. Nanoparticle orientation to control RNA loading and ligand display on extracellular vesicles for cancer regression[J]. Nature Nanotechnology, 2017, 13(1): 82-89.

[151] GUO P. The emerging field of RNA nanotechnology[J]. Nat Nanotechnol, 2010, 5(12): 833-842.